Venous Thromboembolism - Understanding Comorbidities, Approach to Prevention, Injury Impacts, and Endovascular Solutions

Edited by Mojca Božič-Mijovski

Published in London, United Kingdom

Venous Thromboembolism - Understanding Comorbidities, Approach to Prevention, Injury Impacts, and Endovascular Solutions
http://dx.doi.org/10.5772/intechopen.1003312
Edited by Mojca Božič-Mijovski

Contributors
Angélica Araújo Cortines Laxe Renó, Gary J. Curcio, Javier De Miguel Díez, José Javier Jareño Esteban, Jue Wang, Lara Almudena Fernández Bermejo, Leonardo da Cruz Renó, Maria Ángeles Muñoz Lucas, Mostafa A. AL Turk, Oğuzhan Birdal, Parker Wilson, Sergio Campos Téllez, Sidar Şiyar Aydın, William Schwartzman, Zane Gray

First published in London, United Kingdom, 2025 by IntechOpen
IntechOpen is the global imprint of INTECHOPEN LIMITED, registered in England and Wales, registration number: 11086078, 167-169 Great Portland Street, London, W1W 5PF, United Kingdom

For EU product safety concerns: IN TECH d.o.o., Prolaz Marije Krucifikse Kozulić 3, 51000 Rijeka, Croatia, info@intechopen.com or visit our website at intechopen.com.

British Library Cataloguing-in-Publication Data
A catalogue record for this book is available from the British Library

Venous Thromboembolism - Understanding Comorbidities, Approach to Prevention, Injury Impacts, and Endovascular Solutions
Edited by Mojca Božič-Mijovski
p. cm.

This title is part of the Cardiology and Cardiovascular Medicine Book Series, Volume 7
Topic: Cardiovascular Diseases and Health
Series Editor: Kaan Kırali
Topic Editor: Mahi L. Ashwath

Print ISBN 978-0-85466-254-8
Online ISBN 978-0-85466-253-1
eBook (PDF) ISBN 978-0-85466-255-5
ISSN 3033-361X

If disposing of this product, please recycle the paper responsibly.

IntechOpen Book Series

Cardiology and Cardiovascular Medicine

Volume 7

Aims and Scope of the Series

Today, since molecular science on structural causes of oncological pathologies and their molecular treatments are developing at an unbelievable rate, the primary medical cause of death in the twenty-first century will be cardiovascular disease. Neither pandemics that threaten all humanity nor deterioration in the ecosystem will be able to change this fact. Especially, this century seems poised to witness an incredible struggle against atherosclerotic disease, which develops in the arterial walls and results in narrowing and occlusion of the arterial lumen. In addition to this disease, there has been an increasing prevalence of heart rhythm problems, deterioration of heart valves due to aging, and heart failure. Serious vascular pathologies such as stenosis and occlusion, dissection and rupture, and aneurysmal enlargement are also major concerns. Medical and invasive treatment methods may work to save human lives, but they will never provide a real solution. All kinds of medical, technological, and genetic engineering developments obtained in these processes have not yet been sufficient to alleviate or eliminate cardiovascular disease. This book series, Cardiology and Cardiovascular Medicine, includes three topics. The first, Cardiovascular Diseases and Health, reviews important cardiovascular diseases and the developments in their prognosis. The second topic, Cardiovascular Electrophysiology, illuminates the abnormal functioning of the cardiac conduction system, which is caused by all heart pathologies and negatively affects prognosis. The third topic in this series, Cardiovascular Surgery, details treatment for cardiovascular pathologies and how to regulate normal physiological functions with percutaneous or extracorporeal interventions.

Meet the Series Editor

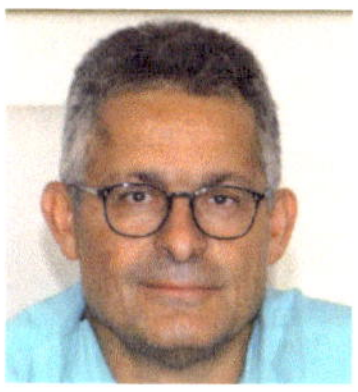

After completing his studies at the Medicine Faculty of Istanbul University in 1990, Prof. Kaan Kırali fulfilled his mandatory medical service and commenced his residency training at Koşuyolu Heart and Research Hospital in 1992. Following five years of assistant education, he pursued further training in England and the USA in 1998. Specializing in laparoscopic and minimally invasive cardiac surgery, he earned the titles of consultant cardiovascular surgeon in 1998, Assistant Professor in 1999, Associate Professor in 2002, and Chief in 2005 at the same hospital. Prof. Kırali also developed an interest in preventive medicine, obtaining an MSc in Public Health from Istanbul University in 2000. Over the past two decades, he has concentrated his scientific pursuits on cardiovascular repairs requiring specialized experience. With his expertise in coronary artery surgery, minimally invasive cardiac surgery, valve repair, and aortic root surgery, he has established new methods for awake coronary bypass revascularization, a new surgical approach for AVR during first and re-operations, aortic valve-sparing procedure, and radiofrequency ablation. Notably, he pioneered awake complete coronary artery bypass grafting (CABG) with bilateral internal mammary arteries (BIMA) and played a crucial role in advancing aortic root surgery with a new aortotomy incision, simplifying aortic valve interventions. Since the year 2000, Prof. Kırali has expanded his interests to heart transplantation, and in recent years, to left ventricular assist devices. He has served as the head of the transplantation department since 2015 and currently continues his work as the director of Koşuyolu High Specialization Education and Research Hospital in Istanbul, Turkey. In his prolific career, he has authored numerous papers in SCI journals, contributed to various book chapters, and served as an editor and reviewer for multiple academic journals. Additionally, he has edited several international books in the field of cardiovascular medicine.

Meet the Volume Editor

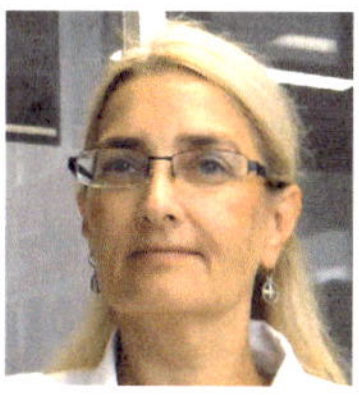

Mojca Božič Mijovski is head of the Laboratory of Hemostasis and Atherothrombosis at the University Medical Centre Ljubljana and assistant professor at the University of Ljubljana. Her research focuses on hemostasis, thrombophilia, and direct oral anticoagulants. As a European specialist in laboratory medicine, she is an active work group member at the European Federation of Clinical Chemistry and Laboratory Medicine. She is also a member of the executive board of the European and Mediterranean League Against Thrombotic Diseases and member of the International Society for Thrombosis and Hemostasis. With numerous publications in high-ranking journals, she has significantly advanced the understanding of thrombosis and anticoagulant therapies.

Contents

Preface **XIII**

Chapter 1 **1**
Comorbidity in Venous Thromboembolic Disease
by José Javier Jareño Esteban, Lara Almudena Fernández Bermejo, Javier De Miguel Díez, Maria Ángeles Muñoz Lucas and Sergio Campos Téllez

Chapter 2 **17**
Deep Vein Thrombosis Prophylaxis for Whom? When?
by Sidar Şiyar Aydın and Oğuzhan Birdal

Chapter 3 **33**
Perspective Chapter: Deep Vein Thrombosis Prevention in Patients with Solid Organ Injuries
by Gary J. Curcio

Chapter 4 **43**
Venous Thromboembolism in Patients with Acute Brain Injury
by Mostafa A. AL Turk

Chapter 5 **55**
Management of Prostate Cancer Associated Disseminated Intravascular Coagulation (DIC): A Multidisciplinary and Individualized Approach
by William Schwartzman, Parker Wilson, Zane Gray and Jue Wang

Chapter 6 **69**
Endovascular Techniques for the Treatment of Venous Diseases
by Leonardo da Cruz Renó and Angélica Araújo Cortines Laxe Renó

Preface

Venous thromboembolism (VTE), which manifests as either deep venous thrombosis (DVT) or pulmonary embolism (PE), is a widespread medical problem that occurs either in isolation or as a complication of other diseases or procedures. It is associated with high morbidity and mortality worldwide and is one of the most common causes of hospitalization [1–3]. Despite its prevalence, there is still much to learn about the pathogenic mechanisms that trigger VTE, how to tailor treatment to the individual risk factors for recurrence, and how to manage VTE in different clinical settings.

This book addresses various aspects of VTE, from common comorbidities in patients with VTE to injury-related VTE, prevention strategies, and innovative treatment techniques. Each chapter comprehensively examines relevant topics that contribute to a deeper understanding of VTE and improve clinical practice.

The book is organized into six chapters. The first chapter deals with various comorbidities associated with VTE. It presents methods and procedures for studying comorbidity in VTE using international registries such as the largest database of patients with VTE, namely RIETE, national registries, specific indexes, and databases of national health systems. In addition, the new concept of the comorbidome, first described by Miguel Divo and colleagues in patients with chronic obstructive pulmonary disease [4], is explained. The comorbidome is a graphical representation of comorbidities' prevalence and risk of death, similar to the solar system. José Javier Jareño and colleagues applied this approach to patients with PE.

This is followed by a chapter on VTE prophylaxis, in which the assessment of thrombosis and bleeding risk in different patient groups is explained, and recommendations and guidelines for prevention management are discussed in detail. Knowing for whom and when to use VTE prophylaxis can significantly reduce avoidable morbidity and mortality. In addition, it is crucial to know which drugs to use in VTE prophylaxis and their dosage. The following chapter deals with a specific patient group: patients with solid organ injuries. It contains a classification system based on the radiological findings of a CT scan, which forms the basis for choosing the appropriate time for initiation and type of prophylaxis, be it mechanical, chemical, or endovascular. Specific recommendations are given for each organ.

Chapter 4 provides comprehensive guidelines for the anticoagulant treatment of patients with neurological injuries who are at particularly high risk of VTE. Prophylaxis and VTE treatment in these patients are challenging, and a tailored approach is essential to optimize outcomes for these patient groups.

Disseminated intravascular coagulation (DIC) is a complex hemostatic disorder that leads to an increased risk of thrombosis and bleeding [5]. Prostate cancer, the most commonly diagnosed cancer in men, can be an underlying cause of DIC [6]. Due to its multifactorial etiology and overlapping clinical features, DIC associated with prostate cancer poses a major challenge for diagnosis and treatment. Chapter 5 provides an overview of epidemiologic data, pathophysiology of DIC in prostate cancer, diagnosis, management, and prognosis. It emphasizes the multidisciplinary and precision medicine approach to optimize outcomes in the face of a complex and difficult condition such as DIC.

The final chapter presents cutting-edge endovascular techniques for treating VTE. Endovascular procedures are more aggressive and are recommended in the acute phase of DVT in patients at high risk of post-thrombotic syndrome and patients with PE associated with hypotension. Various techniques for both DVT and PE are described and illustrated. This chapter is a valuable resource for physicians looking to integrate innovative therapies into their practice.

To summarize, this book is an indispensable resource for healthcare professionals involved in treating VTE. By bringing together diverse perspectives and insights from experts, we aim to promote a deeper understanding of the complexities of VTE and support better patient care. We hope that readers find this collection informative and inspiring as they grapple with the challenges of VTE in their clinical practice.

This preface is intended to engage readers and provide them with an overview of the critical topics covered in this volume on VTE, laying the groundwork for deeper engagement with each chapter.

We want to thank all the authors who have contributed their expertise to this volume and our readers who are committed to advancing knowledge in vascular medicine.

Mojca Božič Mijovski
Department of Vascular Diseases,
University Medical Centre Ljubljana,
Ljubljana, Slovenia

References

[1] Becattini C, Agnelli G. Treatment of venous thromboembolism with new anticoagulant agents. Journal of the American College of Cardiology. 2016;**67**:1941-1955

[2] Hirsh J, Hoak J. Management of deep vein thrombosis and pulmonary embolism. A statement for healthcare professionals. Council on Thrombosis (in consultation with the Council on Cardiovascular Radiology), American Heart Association. Circulation. 1996;**93**:2212-2245

[3] Reitter-Pfoertner S, Waldhoer T, Mayerhofer M, Eigenbauer E, Ay C, Mannhalter C, et al. The influence of thrombophilia on the long-term survival of patients with a history of venous thromboembolism. Thrombosis and Haemostasis. 2013;**109**:79-84

[4] Divo M, Cote C, de Torres JP, Casanova C, Marin JM, Pinto-Plata V, et al. Comorbidities and risk of mortality in patients with chronic obstructive pulmonary disease. American Journal of Respiratory and Critical Care Medicine. 2012;**186**:155-161

[5] Iba T, Helms J, Neal MD, Levy JH. Mechanisms and management of the coagulopathy of trauma and sepsis: trauma-induced coagulopathy, sepsis-induced coagulopathy, and disseminated intravascular coagulation. Journal of Thrombosis and Haemostasis. 2023;**21**:3360-3370

[6] de la Fouchardiere C, Flechon A, Droz JP. Coagulopathy in prostate cancer. The Netherlands Journal of Medicine. 2003;**61**:347-354

Chapter 1

Comorbidity in Venous Thromboembolic Disease

José Javier Jareño Esteban, Lara Almudena Fernández Bermejo, Javier De Miguel Díez, Maria Ángeles Muñoz Lucas and Sergio Campos Téllez

Abstract

Venous thromboembolic disease (VTE) is the third most common vascular disease, immediately after ischemic heart disease and cerebrovascular disease. Its annual incidence is estimated at 1–2 cases 1000 h, but shows a progressive increase with increasing age. Population aging in European Union is one of the main factors related to the increase in VTE. Comorbidity is frequent in the adult population, and chronic diseases, such as chronic obstructive pulmonary disease, idiopathic pulmonary fibrosis, heart failure, etc., have an impact on the prognosis and survival of the individual. Acute VTE is associated with frequent entities (cardiovascular, metabolic, respiratory, psychiatric, etc.). The study of comorbidity in patients with VTE can be performed through different procedures, such as the RIETE registry (Computerized Thromboembolic Disease Registry), an international, multicenter, observational registry, which includes patients with VTE from 2001 to 2024, with more than 100,000 patients included and which includes a registry of comorbidity data. The analysis of codified hospital discharge reports (configuration management database (CMBD)) of the National Health System (NHS) reflects the clinical, sociodemographic, and comorbidity characteristics. Other procedures by means of validated Scores or the Charlson index, and comorbidomes. Cancer and thrombocytosis were the comorbidities mostly related to mortality in VTE.

Keywords: venous thromboembolic, pulmonary embolism, comorbidity, comorbidomes, Charlson index

1. Introduction

Venous thromboembolic disease (VTE) includes two entities, pulmonary embolism (PE) and deep vein thrombosis (DVT). Currently, VTE is a public health problem in the world population and is considered the third most frequent vascular disease in the world, immediately after ischemic heart disease and cerebrovascular disease [1].

Venous thromboembolic disease (VTE) is highly underdiagnosed. The symptoms are not specific and it is necessary to request for different diagnostic tests for confirmation, all of which results in high morbidity and mortality. VTE is responsible for the death of 300.000 people per year in the United States (USA). In the European Union (EU), it was responsible for 370.000 deaths out of a population of 454.4 million people [2].

The estimated number of VTE-related deaths/year in the EU is more than double that of deaths from breast cancer, prostate cancer, AIDS (acquired immunodeficiency syndrome), and traffic accidents combined [3].

The global pandemic by COVID-19, which originated in China in 2019 and in the EU in 2020, has been accompanied by an increased risk of VTE. The estimated global incidence of VTE in patients hospitalized for COVID-19 was 17%. Bleeding events were observed in 8% of patients [4].

There have been few studies in recent years analyzing comorbidity in patients with VTE. Comorbidities are frequent in VTE and have a negative impact on the prognosis and survival of the disease. Studying the different comorbidities, their frequency, presentation, etc., in VTE may be of great interest to improve their treatment and prevention [5].

2. Epidemiology

The annual incidence of VTE in the general population, estimated at about 1–2 cases per 1000 population, has shown an increase in recent decades, varying with age, sex, race, and medical conditions. In the USA, the American Heart Association (AHA) published data on 1.220.000 cases in 2021 [6]. The incidence of VTE in the USA and Canada has increased in recent decades as a result of longer life expectancy in the population and even an increase in diagnostic tests [7]. In Europe, the incidence of VTE in six European countries (for a population of 310.4 million inhabitants) was 296.000 cases of PE and 466.000 cases of DVT. There are no published data concerning the population in Africa (**Table 1**) [8–10].

Population	Incidence
World population	1–2 cases 1000 inhab.
European Union (EU)	PE 296.000 cases–VT 466.000 /310 million inhab.
Argentina	0,7 cases/1000 inhab.
Australia	0,8 cases/1000 inhab.
Asia. South Korea.	0,2 cases/1000 inhab.
USA	115 cases/100.000 inhab.
Africa	No published data

Table 1.
Epidemiology of venous thromboembolic disease (VTE) in the world.

3. Venous thromboembolic disease (VTE): classification

Venous thromboembolic disease (VTE) is an entity whose incidence increases with age, is preventable, and its presentation is related to individual factors, social habits, etc. Obesity and reduced physical activity, among other factors, contribute to increase the risk of VTE.

In epidemiological studies, VTE is often defined and classified as provoked or unprovoked. Provoked events occur at least 3 months prior to the event, such as immobilization, trauma, surgery, cancer, hospitalization, etc. Unprovoked are defined by the absence of these factors. In 2019, the European Society of Cardiology (ESC) and the European Respiratory Society (ERS), in their guidelines for the diagnostic management and treatment of acute pulmonary embolism, discarded the terms provoked and unprovoked [11].

3.1 Comorbidity and VTE

The world's population is aging rapidly, but at the same time, older people are increasing their survival. Aging is accompanied by an increased risk of developing chronic diseases (comorbidities). The risk of developing VTE is higher in the adult and elderly population (**Figure 1**) [12].

Patients with acute VTE present different clinical characteristics from those with arterial cardiovascular disease (ischemic heart disease, acute stroke, etc.). VTE is frequently associated with a number of entities, including neoplastic disease, metabolic disorders, obesity, respiratory disease and, of course, cardiovascular disease, among many other comorbidities. Factors, such as advanced age, aging of the population, surgical interventions, or the use of more aggressive therapies, among many others, influence an increased risk of VTE, as well as its evolution, survival, and mortality [5].

In patients with chronic diseases, such as chronic obstructive pulmonary disease (COPD), asthma, heart failure (HF), or idiopathic pulmonary fibrosis (IPF), comorbidities are frequent and increase with age and disease progression. Their presence has an impact on the prognosis and evolution of the disease [13, 14].

Recently, a new concept has been introduced in the study of comorbidity, syndemia, to describe the concurrence of diseases with shared mechanisms and risk factors [15].

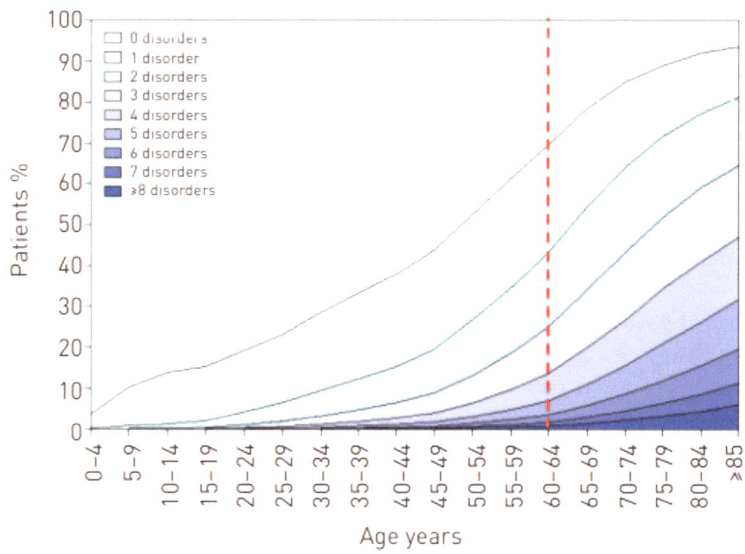

Figure 1.
Number of chronic comorbidities by age stratum. The number of comorbidities increases with age and is larger in individuals 65 years and older. Divo et al. [12].

4. Methodology

Different procedures can be used to study the comorbidities presented by patients with VTE. Clinical trials and scientific publications frequently analyze such comorbidities. The analysis of registries, such as the international RIETE registry or some national registries (SWITER—Switzerland), allows a real approximation of comorbidities in patients with VTE. There are also specific registries, such as the TESEO registry for the oncology population. On the other hand, the study of comorbidity and its implication in survival can be carried out using specific indexes, such as the Charlson index. Finally, studies carried out through the databases of National Health Systems allow analysis of large populations after hospitalization for VTE.

A literature search was carried out in PubMed between 2002 and 2024, using the terms "pulmonary embolism," "deep vein thrombosis," and "comorbidity," published in English or Spanish. We selected publications with randomized studies obtained from national and international registries (**Table 2**).

I - Epidemiological records A - General. • RIETE International Registry • SWITER Registry (Switzerland) • ICOPER (International Cooperative Pulmonary Embolism) Registry • etc. B - Specific. TESEO Registry (VTE in oncology patients) (Spain).
II - Clinical trials
III - Retrospective studies
IV - Studies on patients hospitalized for VTE through the Analysis of the Minimum Basic Data Set (MBDS) of the National Health Systems (Spain)
V- Charlson index
VI - Comorbidome in VTE

Table 2.
Methodology and procedures for the study of comorbidity in venous thromboembolic disease (VTE) [15–19].

5. Epidemiological registries

Registries of patients with VTE are an excellent tool for the analysis of comorbidities. Among the advantages they have over the analysis obtained by other procedures are the absence of limitations with respect to age and the possibility of including different races or ethnicities, marginalized populations, and patients with high comorbidity, who are usually excluded from clinical trials. There are general registries (such as the RIETE [16] and SWITER registry) and specific registries for oncology patients (such as the TESEO registry).

Among the many existing registries, the RIETE registry is worth mentioning because of its size and dissemination. It is an active, international, multicenter, observational registry, with wide dissemination in four continents of the world. The registry, created in our country (Spain) in 2001, has expanded to other countries and continents. Recent publications analyze more than 100.000 patients with VTE from 31 countries and 421 hospitals.

In a recently published study of the registry (RIETE), the differences in adult patients with VTE (>70 years) were analyzed with respect to the younger population (<70 years). It describes the most frequently observed comorbidities: (**Table 3**) [16].

We can observe the differences in comorbidity between the two population groups: in patients older than 70 years old, arterial hypertension, neoplastic disease, diabetes mellitus, respiratory diseases, depression-dementia, and heart failure predominated, in order of frequency. In the younger population (< 70 years old), some differences were observed: arterial hypertension, active cancer, obesity, diabetes mellitus, and respiratory diseases were the most frequently recorded (**Figure 2**).

	Age ≥ 70 years old	**Age ≤ 70 years old**
Cancer	18,9%	20%
Obesity	2,4%	10,1%
Heart failure	10,7%	2,5%
Chronic respiratory disease	14,8%	7,7%
Diabetes mellitus	15,2%	8,2%
Arterial hypertension	48,3%	22,3%
Coronary artery disease	7,2%	2,9%
Stroke	7,3%	2,2%
Peripheral arterial disease	5%	2,3%
Liver disease	0,4%	0,6%
Dementia-Depression	12,2%	4,2%

Modified from García Ortega et al. [16].

Table 3.
Comorbidities in VTE with respect to age (> 70 years old and < 70 years old).

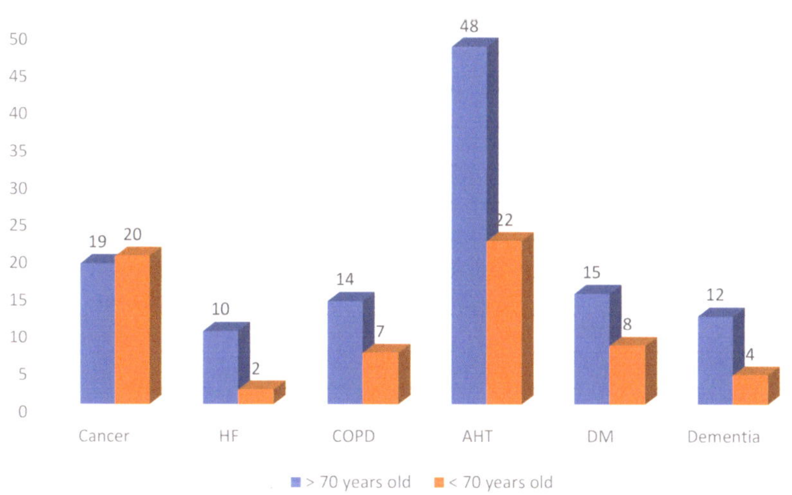

Figure 2.
Most frequent comorbidities in VTE.

6. Studies on patients hospitalized for VTE through analysis of the minimum basic data set (MBDS) of the National Health Systems

The public hospitals of the National Health Systems, through the coded reports on patients hospitalized for PE, have information on the sociodemographic and clinical characteristics, as well as the diagnostic procedures performed on the different patients, allowing an analysis of comorbidity and in-hospital mortality. This is what we call the Minimum Basic Data Set (MBDS).

These retrospective and observational studies have made it possible to analyze over long periods of time (2001–2018) a large sample population of patients hospitalized with Parkinson's disease (PD). On a population of 115.671 patients with PE, an increase in the incidence of PE diagnoses was recorded, from 20.44/100.000 inhabitants in 2002 to 32.69/100.000 inhabitants in 2011, the differences being significant ($p < 0.05$). An increase in comorbidities was also appreciated by Charlson index analysis, being in 2002 (13%) and 20.8% in 2011. Mortality has been decreasing over time, from 12.9% in 2002 to 8.32% in 2011. All this confirms that there has been a change in hospitalizations for PE in recent decades, with an increase in incidence, greater comorbidity, and a decrease in mortality (**Table 4**) [17, 18].

As in the EU, mortality from VTE decreased in the USA and Canada, from 4 to 7 deaths /100.000 h in 2000 to 2–6 deaths/100.000 h in 2017, and this decline was equally observed for both sexes [7].

N = 115,671 patients with VTE	2002	2011	P value
Incidence	20.44	32.69	<0.05
Mortality	12.9%	8.32%	<0.05
Comorbidities (Charlson index)	13.3	20.08	<0.05
Cost per patient	3915€	4372€	<0.05

Table 4.
Trends in hospital admissions for pulmonary embolism in Spain from 2002 to 2011 [14, 15].

6.1 Charlson index

The Charlson comorbidity index allows the prediction of patient mortality by classifying patients by the weight of comorbidities they present. This index evaluates the age of patients and 17 conditions (comorbidities), including cardiovascular, respiratory, neurological, neoplastic, and connective tissue diseases, among others. This is a procedure that, when applied to PD patients with and without cancer, allows us to analyze the differences in comorbidities and their impact on survival [19–22].

There are not many studies that analyze the Charlson index and comorbidity in PE patients. The Danish study by Ording et al., which compared 62.376 patients with breast cancer versus 304.803 people without breast cancer in the general population, found little relationship between breast cancer and the Charlson index in the rate of VTE [23]. The results published by Fernandez et al. in 2021 [19], in a population of 308 patients with PE, 108 of them with PE and cancer, confirmed that the mean Charlson index in patients with PE and cancer was higher than in those with PE without cancer (7,2 vs. 4,5, respectively). Likewise, patients with a Charlson index above 5 had a 10 times higher risk of death than those with a Charlson index of 0 ($p = 0.0019$). Patients with PE and cancer had a higher risk of death and higher mortality 30 days and 1 year after the episode, compared to those with PE without cancer, with significant differences in survival ($p < 0.001$) (**Figures 3** and **4**).

The Charlson index is a useful tool in the study of comorbidities in patients with VTE and cancer and is an independent risk factor related to mortality [24]. In the paper published by Hira Shahzad [25], VTE occurred in 17.9% of patients with lung cancer, the mean Charlson index in patients with VTE was 7,4 + 3,2, compared to 6,5 + 2,5 in patients without VTE. On correlation analysis, a significant correlation was found between Charlson index and the occurrence of VTE.

Likewise, the Charlson index helps to predict whether there is a higher short- and long-term mortality in patients with PE [5, 19]. In an Australian study including 1023 patients diagnosed with VTE and stratifying them into Charlson index 0 and Charlson index ≥1, 34% had an in-hospital mortality of 0 with in-hospital mortality in this group of only 0,3, similar to that of the general population [26]. The Charlson index has good discriminatory power to predict in-hospital and long-term events after a VTE event [26]. Increased comorbidity analyzed by the Charlson index is associated with increased mortality (**Figures 3** and **4**) [19] and patients with VTE and cancer have greater comorbidity assessed by the Charlson index compared to patients with VTE without cancer [19, 21, 27], with the Charlson index being an independent risk factor associated with mortality.

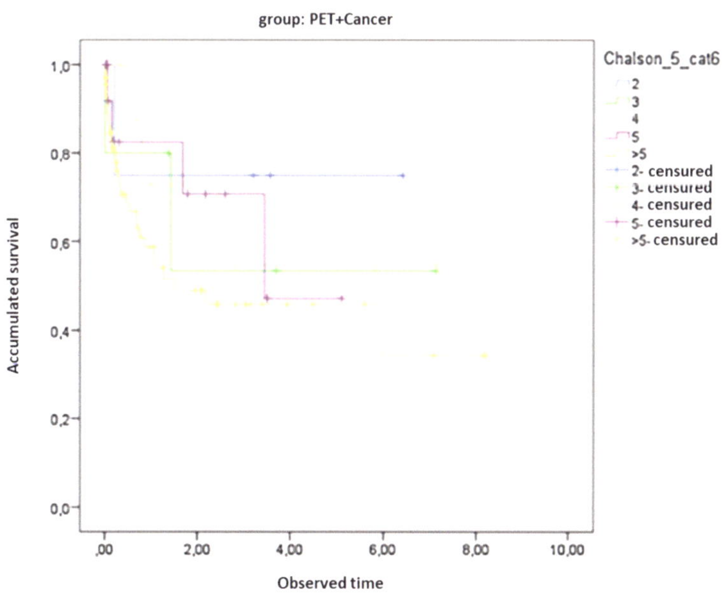

Figure 3.
Representation of the survival of patients with VTE and cancer according to the categorized Charlson index. Kaplan-Meier survival curve. Modified from Fernandez et al. [19].

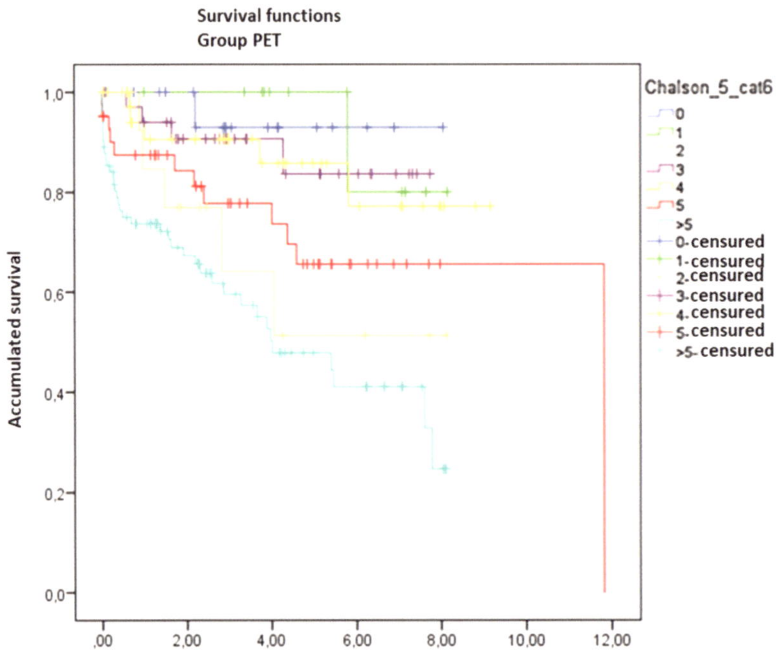

Figure 4.
Representation of survival of patients with VTE without cancer as a function of the categorized Charlson index. Kaplan-Meier survival curve. Modified from Fernandez et al. [19].

7. Comorbidome

The study of comorbidities in chronic respiratory diseases, such as COPD, through new indexes, such as the COTE index, together with the graphical representation of prevalence and its impact on mortality, was developed by DIVO et al. in 2012 in COPD patients. Imitating the solar system, the different comorbidities in order of prevalence and according to their repercussions on mortality (proximity to the orbital center) are placed in the different orbits, visually representing what we know as comorbidome [28, 29]. Subsequently, new publications have appeared with representation of comorbidities and comorbidome in patients with idiopathic pulmonary fibrosis (IPF) [29].

The study of the different comorbidities in recent publications in patients with PD from the RIETE registry has allowed us to know their different prevalences, as well as their impact on mortality. The development of a comorbidome in PE is not known, therefore we believe that it is an opportunity for its development [6, 10, 11].

In the PE comorbidome (**Figure 5**), the most frequently recorded comorbidities are represented. Active cancer represents the comorbidity most related to mortality (OR > 5), due to its proximity to the center of the orbit (death); it is followed by thrombopenia (OR > 2). Other comorbidities are placed at a distance from these, with less impact on mortality: liver disease (OR > 1), heart failure (OR > 1), anemia (OR > 1), depression (OR > 1), and COPD (OR > 1). Finally, arterial hypertension showed a high prevalence but little relationship with mortality (OR=0,78) [30].

DOI: http://dx.doi.org/10.5772/intechopen.1006537

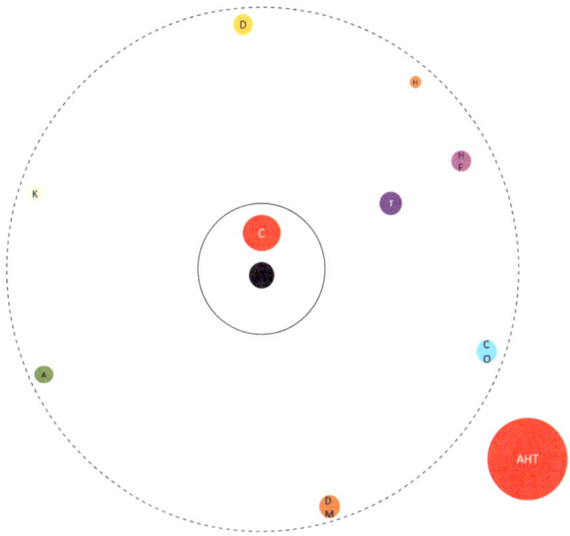

COMORBIDITIES - VTE	OR
CANCER (C)	5
THROMBOPENIA (T)	2,69
HEPATIC DISEASE (H)	1,94
CKD (K)	1,89
HF (HF)	1,69
ANEMIA (A)	1,62
DEPRESSION (D)	1,51
COPD (CO)	1,37
DM	1,26
AHT	0,79

Figure 5.
Comorbidome in PE. Representation of the most frequent comorbidities and their impact on mortality [16, 17].

8. Most frequent comorbidities related to VTE

8.1 Cancer

Thromboembolic complications are a common event in patients with cancer and one of the main causes of morbidity and mortality [31]. Cancer is present in more than 20% of patients with VTE. VTE is the second cause of death in patients with neoplasia [32]. Active cancer increases the risk of VTE approximately 4 to 7 times compared to the general population [33, 34].

Venous thromboembolic disease (VTE) may precede the diagnosis of a neoplasm by months or years. It is estimated that in around 2–12% of VTE cases is the first manifestation of an occult cancer 31. However, VTE is more frequently present once the patient has been diagnosed, throughout the course of the disease. Up to 88% of thrombotic events present with these characteristics [35, 36].

According to Chew et al. [37], metastatic disease at the time of diagnosis is the greatest predictor of VTE, with the risk of developing it being 4 to 13 times greater than in patients with localized disease. The highest incidence in patients with metastatic disease was observed in cancer of the pancreas, stomach, bladder, uterus, kidney, and lung [37]. The risk of presenting a VTE in patients with cancer is highest in the first 3 months after diagnosis, is somewhat lower during the following 3–12 months, and is low in the following 2 and 3 years [38].

The incidence of VTE varies depending on the type of cancer [39]. The tumors that have been associated with the highest risk of developing a thromboembolic event are pancreatic cancer (14%) and brain tumors (11%). The following tumors correspond to chronic myeloid leukemia (7.4%), stomach cancer (7.4%), esophagus (5.8%), kidney (4.3%), and lung (4.3%). Breast and prostate cancers have a low incidence (0.1 and 0.9%) [39, 40].

9. Hematological disorders: thrombophilia, thrombocytopenia, and neutropenia

Various hematological alterations have been related to the appearance of VTE. Thrombophilias are the best known, well related to hematological disorders, neoplasias, idiopathic causes, etc.

In the study by Merkow et al. [41], the presence of thrombocytosis (>400.000 platelets/microl) in patients undergoing oncological surgery constitutes a risk factor for the development of VTE, increasing the probability of its presentation by 1.6% beyond the month of the intervention, which advises extending thromboprophylactic therapies in patients undergoing surgery for cancer [42, 43].

Among all these alterations, thrombocytopenia was the alteration most related to mortality due to VTE.

Other hematological alterations, such as neutropenia, have been related to thromboembolic episodes. In a retrospective study of 66.106 cancer patients admitted for neutropenia, between 2,74 and 12,1% presented a thromboembolic event [44].

9.1 Other comorbidities

There are comorbidities such as hypertension and DM that are very common among the general population, and therefore among patients with VTE, but their presence does not correlate with mortality. In **Figure 4**, both comorbidities appear in the outermost orbits, far from the center of mortality in the comorbidome. Similar characteristics with hypertension and DM occur in other chronic diseases, such as COPD and IPF [28, 29, 30].

10. Conclusions

i. Venous thromboembolic disease (VTE) is a very prevalent, underdiagnosed entity, associated with high mortality. Its incidence is increasing in the world with the use of better diagnostic procedures.

ii. Comorbidities in VTE are frequent, with cancer being one of the most prominent (20–30%).

iii. The identification of comorbidities accompanying VTE may help to improve prognosis and survival.

iv. The Charlson index and the elaboration of comorbidome can be useful in the identification of comorbidities with prognostic implication in VTE.

Author details

José Javier Jareño Esteban[1*], Lara Almudena Fernández Bermejo[2*],
Javier De Miguel Díez[3], Maria Ángeles Muñoz Lucas[4] and Sergio Campos Téllez[1]

1 Pneumology Central University Hospital of the Defense, Madrid, Spain

2 Internal Medicine, Thrombosis Unit, Santa Barbara Hospital, Ciudad Real, Spain

3 Pneumology Hospital General Universitario Gregorio Marañon, Madrid, Spain

4 Teaching Department, Central Hospital of the Defense, Madrid, Spain

*Address all correspondence to: jjjarenoesteban@yahoo.es
and larafernandezber@gmail.com

References

[1] Beckman MG, Hooper WC, Critchley SE, Ortel TL. Venous thromboembolism: A public health concern. American Journal of Preventive Medicine. 2010;**38**(Suppl. 4):495. DOI: 10.1016/j.amepre.2009.12.017

[2] Cohen AT, Agnelli G, Anderson FA, Arcelus JI, Bergqvist D, Brecht JG, et al. Tromboembolismo venoso (TEV) en Europa. El número de eventos de TEV y la morbilidad y mortalidad asociadas. Thromb Haesmost. 2007;**98**:756-764

[3] Lobo JL, Alonso S, Arenas J, Doménech P, Escribano P, Fernández Capitán C, et al. Multidisciplinary consensus for the management of pulmonary thromboembolism. Consenso multidisciplinar Para el manejo de la tromboembolia de pulmón. Archivos de Bronconeumología. 2022;**58**:246-254. DOI: 10.1016/j. arbres2021.01.031

[4] Jiménez D, García-Sánchez A, Rali P, Muriel A, Bikdeli B, Ruiz-Artacho P, et al. Incidence of VTE and bleeding among hospitalized patients with coronavirus disease 2019. A systematic review and meta-analysis. Chest. 2021;**159**:1182-1196

[5] Jareño JJ, De Miguel J, Fernández LA. Pulmonary embolism and comorbidity. Open Respiratory Archives. 2022;**4**:100188. DOI: 10.1016/j. oprest.2022.100188

[6] Bikdeli B, Wang Y, Jimenez D, Parikh SA, Monreal M, Goldhaber SZ, et al. Pulmonary embolism hospitalization, readmission, and mortality rates in US older adults 1995-2015. Journal of the American Medical Association. 2019;**322**:574-576. DOI: 10.1001/jama.2019.8594

[7] Barco S, Valerio L, Cohen A, Goldhaber S, Hunt B, Jimenez D, et al. Age-sex specific pulmonary embolism-related mortality in the USA and Canada and of the CDC multiple cause of death database. The Lancet Respiratory Medicine. 2021;**9**:33-42

[8] Lutsey SPL, Zakai N. Epidemiology and prevention of venous thromboembolism. Nature Reviews. Cardiology. 2023;**20**:248-262. DOI: 10.1038/s41569-00787

[9] Freund Y, Cohen-Aubart F, Bloom B. Acute pulmonary embolism: A review. JAMA. 2022;**328**:1336-1345. DOI: 10.1001/jama.2022.16815

[10] López Jiménez L, Montero M, González Fajardo JA, Arcelus JL, Suárez C, Lobo JL, et al. Venous thromboembolism in very elderly patients: Findings a prospective registry (RIETE). Haematologica. 2006;**91**:1046-1051

[11] Konstantinides SV, Meyer G, Becattini C, Bueno H, Geersing GJ, Harjola VP, et al. ESC guidelines for the diagnosis and management of acute pulmonary embolism developed in collaboration with the ERS: The task force for the diagnosis and management of acute pulmonary embolism of the ESC. European Respiratory Journal. 2019;**54**(3):1901647. DOI: 10.1183/13993003.01647-2019

[12] Divo MJ, Martinez C, Mannino D. Ageing and the epidemiology of multimorbidity. The European Respiratory Journal. 2014;**44**:1055-1068. DOI: 10.1183/09031936.00059814

[13] Friz HP, Orenti A, Gelfi E, Motto E, Primitz L, d'Oro LC, et al. Predictors

of medium- and long-term mortality in elderly patients with acute pulmonary embolism. Heliyon. 2020;**6**:e04857

[14] Chan TF, Ngian VJJ, Hsu K, Frankel A, Ong BS. Pulmonary embolism: Clinical presentation and diagnosis in the oldest old. Internal Medicine Journal. 2020;**50**:627-631

[15] Fabri L, Celli B, Agusti A, Criner G, Dransfield M, Divo M, et al. COPD and multimorbidity: Recognizing and addressing a syndemic occurrence. The Lancet Respiratory Medicine. 2023;**11**:1020-1034. DOI: 10.1016/52213-2600(23)00261-8

[16] Ortega AG, Jiménez D, Pedro-Tudela A, Pérez-Ductor C, Fernández-Capitán C, Falgá C, et al. Diferencias relacionadas con la edad en la presentación, el tratamiento y los resultados clínicos de 100.000 pacientes con tromboembolismo venoso en el registro RIETE. 2024;**60**(3):143-152. DOI: 10.1016/j.arbres.2023.12.016

[17] De Miguel DJ, Albaladejo Vicente R, López de Andres A, Hernández Barrera V, Jiménez D, Monreal M, et al. Changing trends in hospital admissions for pulmonary embolism in Spain from 2001 to 2018. Journal of Clinical Medicine. 2020;**9**:3221

[18] De Miguel DJ, Jiménez Garcia R, Jiménez D, Monreal M, Guijarro R, Otero R, et al. Trends in hospital admissions for pulmonary embolism in Spain from 2002 to 2011. The European Respiratory Journal. 2014;**44**:942-950

[19] Fernández Bermejo LA, Gútierrez Ortega C, Jareño EJ. Valor pronóstico del índice de Charlson en la mortalidad en pacientes con embolia pulmonar asociada a cáncer frente a embolia pulmonar no tumoral. Medicina Clinica. 2022;**158**:201-5. DOI: 10.1016/j.medcli.2021.02.007

[20] Golpe R, Pérez de Llano LA, Castro-Aañón O. Prognostic of the Charlson comorbidity index in pulmonary embolism. Respiration. 2013;**85**:438

[21] Zhou C, Wang YX, Zhong X, Yang ZH, Zhang M, Zhou HX, et al. Risk factors associated with mortality in patient with non-high-risk pulmonary embolism and cancer and the prognostic value of Charlson comorbidity index. Zhonghua Yi Xue Za Zhi. 2020;**100**:2383-2387

[22] Zhou H, Tang Y, Wang L, Shi C, Feng Y, Yi Q. Risk factors associated with long-term mortality in patients with pulmonary embolism and the predictive value of Charlson comorbidity index. Zhonghua Yi, Xue Za Zhi. 2016;**96**:273-276

[23] Ording AG, Horváth-Puhó E, Garne JP, et al. Impact of comorbidity on risk of venous thromboembolism in patients with breast cancer: A Danish population-based cohort study. BMJ Open. 2014;**4**:e005082

[24] Truonh AH, Lio UK, Shah A, Arshdad H, Patel P, Wang Y, et al. Charlson comorbidity index predicts readmission risk following acute pulmonary embolism hospitalization. Chest. 2023;**17**:164

[25] Shahzad H. Charlson comorbidity index and VTE in lung cancer. Chest. 2017. DOI: 10.1016/j.chest.2017.08.673

[26] Ng AC, Chow V, Yong AS, Chung T, Kritharides L. Prognostic impact of the Charlson comorbidity index on mortality following acute pulmonary embolism. Respiration. 2013;**85**(5):408-416

[27] Divo M, Cote C, De Torres JP, et al. Comorbidities and risk of mortality in patients with COPD. American Journal of

Respiratory and Critical Care Medicine. 2012;**186**:155-161

[28] Almagro P, Cabrera FJ, Diez J, et al. Comorbilidades y pronóstico a corto plazo en pacientes hospitalizados por exacerbación aguda de EPOC: el estudio EPOC en Servicios de medicina interna (ESMI). Chest. 2012;**142**(5):1126-1133. DOI: 10.1378/Chest.11-2413

[29] Kreuter M, Ehlers-Tenenbaum S, Palmowski K, Bruhwyler J, Oltmanns U, Muley R, et al. Impact of comorbidities on mortality in patients with idiopathic pulmonary fibrosis. PLoS One. 2016;**11**(3):E0151425. DOI: 10.1371/journal.pone.0151425

[30] Tafur A, Fuentes H, Caprini JA, Rivas A, Uresandi F, Duce R, et al. Predictors of early mortality in cancer-associated thrombosis: Analysis of the RIETE database. TH Open. 2018;**2**:e158-e166

[31] Khorana AA, Francis CW, Culakowa E, Kuderer NM, Lyman GH. Thromboembolism is a leading cause of death patients receiving outpatient chemotherapy. Journal of Thrombosis and Haemostasis. 2007;**5**:632-634

[32] Prandoni P, Falanga A, Piciolli A. Cancer and venous thromboembolism. The Lancet Oncology. 2005;**6**:401-410

[33] Dallah S, Wan JY, Nguyen NP. Venous thrombosis in patients with solid tumors: Determination of frequency and characteristics. Thrombosis and Haemostasis. 2002;**87**:575-579

[34] Heit JA, O'Fallon WM, Petterson TM, Lohse CM, Silverstein MD, Mohr DN, et al. Relative impact of the risk for deep vein thrombosis and pulmonary embolism: A population-based study. Archives of Internal Medicine. 2002;**162**:1245-1248

[35] Epstein AS, Ga Soff M, Capanu CC, Shah MA, Kelsen DP, et al. Analysis of incidence and clinical outcomes in patients with thromboembolic events and invasive exocrine pancreatic cancer. Cancer. 2012;**118**:3053-3061

[36] Wun T, White RH. Epidemiology of cancer related venous thromboembolism. Best Practice & Research. Clinical Haematology. 2009;**22**:9-23

[37] Chew HK, Wun T, Harvey D, Zhou H, White RH. Incidence of venous thromboembolism and its effect on survival among patients with common cancers. Archives of Internal Medicine. 2006;**166**(4):458-464

[38] Blom JW, Doggen CJ, Osanto S, Rosendaal FR. Malignancies, prothrombotic mutations, and the risk venous thrombosis. JAMA. 2005;**293**:715-722

[39] Ku GH, White RH, Chew HK, Harvey DJ, Zhou H, Wun T. Venous thromboembolism in patients with acute leukemia. Incidence, risk factors, and effect on survival. Blood. 2009;**113**:3911-3917

[40] Khorana AA, Rao MV. Approaches to risk-stratifying cancer patients for venous thromboembolism. Thrombosis Research. 2007;**120**(Suppl. 2):S41-S50

[41] Merkow RP, Bilimoria KY, MacCarter MD, et al. Post-discharge venous thromboembolism after cancer surgery: Extending the case for extended prophylaxis. Annals of Surgery. 2011;**254**:131

[42] Khorana AA. Venous thromboembolism prevention in cancer outpatients. Journal of the National Comprehensive Cancer Network. 2013;**11**:1431

[43] Fernández Bermejo L, Jareño JJ, De Miguel DJ, Dominguez IM, Gónzalez C, Ochoa P. Evaluation of the Khorana predictive thrombotic risk and Thromboprophylaxis score in cancer patients in a third level hospital. Open Respiratory Archives. 2022;**4**:100170

[44] Khorana AA, Francis CW, Culakova E, Fisher RJ, Kuderer NM, Lyman GH. Thromboembolism in hospitalized neutropenic cancer patients. Journal of Clinical Oncology. 2006;**24**:484-490

Chapter 2

Deep Vein Thrombosis Prophylaxis for Whom? When?

Sidar Şiyar Aydın and Oğuzhan Birdal

Abstract

Deep vein thrombosis (DVT) is a type of thrombus seen in the deep leg veins. DVT is a clinical condition that can cause pulmonary embolism. Pulmonary embolism is a significant contributor to the rates of illness and death worldwide. In a healthy state, blood circulation is regulated by procoagulant and anticoagulant factors to prevent the formation of blood clots. However, conditions called Virchow's triad, whose components are hypercoagulation, venous stasis, and endothelial damage, increase the tendency to DVT if one or more of these components are present. Using prophylaxis is recommended for preventing DVT in patients with predisposing conditions. Prophylaxis reduces morbidity and mortality. Conditions such as immobility, orthopedic surgery, obesity, advanced age, active cancer, and hormone replacement therapy may increase the risk of venous thrombosis. Those patients who present with multiple risk factors are identified as being at high risk for DVT and are administered prophylactic anticoagulants.

Keywords: anticoagulants agents, deep vein thrombosis, prophylaxis, pulmonary embolism, thromboembolism

1. Introduction

Deep venous thrombosis (DVT) is a thrombus in the body's deep veins. Although the underlying cause varies from patient to patient, damage to the vein wall, venous stasis, and increased procoagulant activity (Virchow triad) have been blamed for its underlying pathophysiology. DVT and associated pulmonary thromboembolism (PE) can cause preventable morbidity and mortality [1, 2]. DVT is seen at a rate of 0.05–0.1% in the general flow [3]. However, this rate is higher in patients with predisposing causes or hospitalization. The incidence of DVT varies depending on the person, gender, race, and predisposing conditions. The incidence of DVT doubles with every 10-year increase in age [4]. DVT is more common in men of all age groups when predisposing factors such as hormonal and oral contraceptive use specific to women are excluded [5]. While Africans have a higher incidence of DVT, Asians have a lower incidence of DVT. Even the seasons can adjust the appearance of DVT—for example, the incidence of DVT increases in winter months [6]. Although DVT can be seen without any risk factors, it can also be seen as a result of provocation by unprovoked hereditary and acquired risk factors. Acquired risk factors are more common than hereditary ones. Acquired risk factors include cancer, obesity, acute medical illness,

IntechOpen

major surgery or trauma, immobility (usually inpatients and for at least 3 days), pregnancy, hormone replacement therapy, inflammatory disease, antiphospholipid syndrome, prolonged passive travel, and seated immobility syndrome, which can occur with increased interest in computer games [7]. The main hereditary risk factor is the non-O blood group, which doubles the risk of occurrence in venous thromboembolism (VTE) [8]. Also among the hereditary risk factors are homozygous and heterozygous factors such as V Leiden mutation, thrombophilia due to antithrombin, and protein C or S deficiency [9].

Application of DVT prophylaxis in a specific patient population reduces the rate of VTE and its associated morbidity and mortality. DVT prophylaxis should be applied to patients undergoing thoracic surgery, spinal and cranial surgery, hip fracture surgery, knee surgery, urological and cancer surgery, and significant trauma patients. At the same time, even if surgery is not performed, some hospitalized patient groups are candidates for VTE prophylaxis. Patients over 60 years of age with at least one risk factor for DVT, ischemic stroke patients, patients with a history of venous thromboembolism, patients with acute and chronic lung disease, decompensated heart failure patients, acute inflammatory disease, sepsis, active cancer, and antenatal patients those with more than three obstetric risks should receive VTE prophylaxis [10]. DVT prophylaxis is applied to these patient groups for a certain period. Generally, low molecular weight Heparin (LMWH) is preferred for prophylaxis. This book section will discuss which patient groups will be given VTE prophylaxis and for how long.

2. Risk factors for DVT

Many hereditary or acquired risk factors may affect Virchow's triad, which is accused in the pathogenesis of DVT (**Table 1**). Malignancy, patients undergoing surgery, smoking, heart failure, inflammatory disease, and previous VTE are the main acquired risk factors. Acquired factors are relatively more straightforward to detect by a physician [11]. However, detecting hereditary risk factors can be challenging. Although this situation is challenging for the physician, careful anamnesis, physical examination, and laboratory tests facilitate the detection of acquired and hereditary risk factors [12].

Acquired factors	Hereditary factors
Advanced Age	Factor V Leiden Mutation
immobility	Protein C and S deficiency
Cigarette	Antithrombin Deficiency
Cancer	Antiphospholipid Syndrome
Heart Failure	Sickle Cell Anemia
Trauma	Family History of Thrombophilia
Surgical History	Prothrombin Mutations
Presence of Central Catheter	
Pregnancy	
Oral Contraceptive Use	
Obesity	
Previous DVT History	

Table 1.
Risk factors for VTE.

Low-risk group	Medium risk group	High-risk group
Surgical procedures that take less than 30 minutes Laparoscopic surgeries Obesity Smoke Having Varicose Veins Immobility Lasting Less Than 3 Days	Thrombophilia Heart Failure Oral Contraceptive Use Pregnancy Major Surgery (not exceeding 7 days) Infection requiring Intravenous treatment Immobility lasting more than 3 days	Pelvis or Long Bone FractureS Ischemic Stroke Trauma Neurosurgery Malignancy Postoperative Intubation

Table 2.
Risk classification for VTE.

Risk factors should be evaluated, especially in hospitalized patients scheduled for surgery or medical treatment. According to risk factors, patients can be classified as low, medium, and high in terms of VTE (**Table 2**) [13]. Chemoprophylaxis can be started in patients according to risk assessment, which will minimize the risk of VTE.

3. Assessment of bleeding risk

The VTE-BLEED risk score is a bleeding risk score assessment derived from a post hoc analysis of the RE-COVER study. It is based on the presence of cancer, hypertension, anemia, bleeding history, age, and renal functions. While patients with a score below two were considered to be at low risk for bleeding, patients with a score of 2 or higher were considered to be at high risk (**Table 3**). Patients at high risk of bleeding face a 5-fold increased risk of bleeding with anticoagulant use compared to low-risk groups. If the probability of bleeding is higher than the probability of developing VTE, anticoagulation can be avoided in these patient groups [14].

Factor	Score
Active Cancer[1]	2
Man with Uncontrolled Hypertension[2]	1
Anemia[3]	1.5
Bleeding History[4]	1.5
Age ≥ 60	1.5
Renal Dysfunction[5]	1.5
Classification of patients according to VTE-BLEED score	
Low Risk of Bleeding High Bleeding Risk	Total score < 2 Total score ≥ 2

[1]*Receiving a diagnosis of cancer within 6 months before VTE diagnosis.*
[2]*Uncontrolled hypertension, basal systolic blood pressure 140 mmHg.*
[3]*Hemoglobin <13 g/dL for men, Hemoglobin <12 g/dL for women.*
[4]*Previous major or non-major bleeding, rectal bleeding, frequent nosebleeds, hematuria.*
[5]*Estimated glomerular filtration rate (eGFR) is defined as <60 ml/min (eGFR calculated with the Cockcroft-Gaults formula).*

Table 3.
VTE-BLEED score.

4. VTE prophylaxis in patient groups

Among the risk groups for VTE, cancer, surgical patients, trauma patients, pregnant women, and immobile patients have an important place. Tendency to thrombosis and immobility, which occur through various mechanisms in these patient groups, pose a severe risk for VTE [15]. It is clinically essential to thoroughly examine this patient group and determine which population should receive VTE prophylaxis and for how long. In this section, we discussed the evaluation of this group of patients in terms of VTE prophylaxis.

4.1 Cancer patients

Recent studies have shown that the incidence of VTE in cancer patients has increased approximately three times. This situation has increased hospitalization rates and caused increases in treatment costs [16]. The incidence of VTE varies depending on the cancer location. While this rate is 8.2% in bladder cancer, it can be seen in 19.2% in pancreatic cancer [17]. Considering the VTE risk in this patient group, a scoring system developed by Khorana is used, and many guidelines approve it [18, 19]. The ONCOTHROMB score is another score that has recently been used to evaluate cancer patients for VTE prophylaxis [20]. A study even compares it with the Khorana score [21]. However, we found it appropriate to give the Khona score, which has been used for many years, in this section. Khrona scoring system is based on the location of cancer, platelet, and leukocyte count before chemotherapy, hemoglobin level, and body mass index. Scoring three or more is classified as high risk, 1–2 as medium risk, and 0 points as low risk. Details about the scoring system are given in **Table 4**.

High-risk patients who do not have contraindications to anticoagulant use should be started on anticoagulants and/or intermittent pneumatic devices, and graduated compression stockings should be applied. If there are any contraindications to using anticoagulants, intermittent pneumatic devices and/or graduated compression stockings can be applied. Cancer patients who undergo surgery should use anticoagulant treatment for about one month after discharge. However, medical oncology patients who have not undergone surgery are at high risk for VTE if they are diagnosed with multiple myeloma and are using lenalidomide or thalidomide at discharge. In this patient group, 40 mg LMWH or warfarin (international normalized ratio: 2–3)

Patient characteristics	Risk Skoru
Cancer Localization	
Stomach and pancreatic cancer	2
Lung, Lymphoma, Gynecological, Bladder, Testicular	1
Platelet count before chemotherapy $\geq 350 \times 10^9/L$	1
Hemoglobin <10 g/dL or using red blood cell growth factor	1
Leukocyte count before chemotherapy $>11 \times 10^9/L$	1
Body mass index ≥ 35 kg/m^2	1
If the total Score is ≥3, it is high risk, if the total Score is 1–2, it is medium risk, and if the total Score is 0, it is low risk.	

Table 4.
Risk scoring for VTE in cancer patients.

should be used daily. While acetylsalicylic acid 81–325 mg once a day is recommended for VTE prophylaxis in low-risk myeloma patients after discharge, routine VTE prophylaxis is not recommended for the remaining patients with cancer (who have not undergone surgery) [22].

4.2 VTE prophylaxis in surgical patients

Although many scoring systems are used to determine the risk of VTE in surgical patients, the Caprini score is one of the most widely used [23]. The Caprini score was developed in 2005 and tested and validated to determine the risk of VTE in most surgical patients [13, 24–26]. The European Society of Hematology VTE prophylaxis guideline for perioperative patients recommends using the Caprini score [27]. Caprini score classifies patients into three groups due to the evaluation of approximately 37–40 parameters. Patients with a total score of 0–4 are classified as low risk, patients with a score of 5–8 as medium risk, and patients with a total score of ≥9 as high risk. Caprini score parameters and scoring details are given in **Table 5**. New risk scores were added to the Caprini score as a result of research conducted after it was first published, and sometimes, there were changes in the score distribution [28]. However, studies similar to the first version could not confirm updates after the first version. In fact, one study showed that the new version performed worse in some surgical patients than the first version [29]. For this reason, we deemed it appropriate to share the first version published in 2005 in this section.

1 Point for Each Risk Factor Age 41–60 Planned minor surgery Major surgery performed within one month Varicose veins History of inflammatory bone disease Recurrent leg swelling Obesity Acute myocardial infarction Congestive heart failure Sepsis within one month Lung disease, including pneumonia, within one month Chronic obstructive pulmonary disease Medical patients on bed rest	**2 Points for Each Risk Factor** Age between 60 and 74 Arthroscopic surgery Malignancy Major surgery (lasting >45 minutes) Laparoscopic surgery (lasting >45 minutes) Patients on bed rest for more than 72 hours Being in an immobile cast within one month Central venous access **5 Points for Each Risk Factor** Elective major lower extremity arthroscopy Hip, pelvis, or leg fracture within one month stroke within one month Multiple trauma within one month Acute spinal trauma accompanied by paralysis within one month
3 Points for Each Risk Factor ≥75 years old History of PTE/DVT Family history of thrombosis Positive Factor V Leiden Prothrombin 20210A mutation Serum homocysteine elevation Positive lupus anticoagulant Anticardiolipin antibody elevation Heparin-induced thrombocytopenia Other acquired and inherited thrombophilias	**1 Point for Each Risk Factor (For women only)** Oral contraceptive or hormone replacement therapy Pregnancy or postpartum (<1 month) History of unexplained stillborn baby, recurrent spontaneous miscarriage (≥3), premature birth with toxemia, or history of growth-restricted baby

Table 5.
Caprini risk score.

Various agents are commonly used for VTE prophylaxis in surgical patients. Acetylsalicylic acid has been used for VTE prophylaxis in total knee and hip replacement surgeries and hip fracture operations. However, the dose margin varies between 75 mg and 1300 mg in studies. Additionally, the duration of use for VTE prophylaxis varied between two days and six weeks [30]. Low-dose unfractionated heparin is another agent used in VTE prophylaxis. A dose of 5000 IU has been recommended for most surgical procedures every 8–12 hours. It should be started 2 hours before the surgical procedure. 5000 IU should be administered once every 12 hours in orthopedic surgical procedures, starting 12 hours before/after the operation [31]. In high-risk surgeries such as cancer surgery, 5000 IU should be started 2 hours before the procedure and administered once every 8 hours [32]. LMWH is the most common agent used in VTE prophylaxis. In abdominal surgeries, Enoksaparin 40 mg/day should be administered and should be started 2–12 hours before the surgical procedure. In total hip and knee replacement procedures, 30 mg should be administered once every 12 hours and started 12 hours before or 12 hours after the operation. A daily dosage of 40 mg is recommended for hip fracture operations. For other surgical procedures, 40 mg/day should be administered 10–12 hours before the operation [32, 33]. Fondaparinux is another agent used for VTE prophylaxis. However, it is not used in abdominal surgeries, total knee and hip prostheses, or hip fracture operations.

A postoperative dosage of 2.5 mg daily has been suggested for other surgical procedures. This medication should be avoided in patients with a creatinine clearance of less than 30 ml/min and a body weight of less than 50 kg [34]. Additionally, Factor Xa inhibitors are a practical option for VTE prophylaxis in surgical patients. For total hip and knee replacement surgeries, apixaban 2.5 mg should be taken every 12 hours, starting 12–24 hours after the surgery, and rivaroxaban 10 mg should be taken once a day, starting 6–10 hours after the surgery. There is no data on the use of edoxaban in total knee replacement operations. For other surgical procedures, 30 mg/day is recommended 6–24 hours after surgery. However, there is more clinical experience using rivaroxaban and apixaban for VTE prophylaxis in surgical patients [35].

4.3 Trauma patients

The incidence of DVT in trauma patients can be seen between 5 and 63%, depending on the risk factors of the patients, the prophylaxis methods applied, and the choice of diagnostic techniques [36, 37]. Many factors can affect the development of post-traumatic VTE. Reasons such as depletion of coagulation factors, acidosis, hypothermia, hemodilution caused by the administration of intravenous fluids and blood products, immobility, and activation of fibrinolytic pathways due to shock or anticoagulant use have been suggested [38]. Greenfield and colleagues examined risk factors and developed the risk assessment profile (RAP) to determine the incidence of DVT in trauma patients [39]. Patients with an RAP score of 5 or higher are three times more likely to develop DVT compared to those with an RAP score of less than 5 [40]. The RAP scoring details are clearly outlined in **Table 6**.

There are some points to consider when starting thromboprophylaxis in a trauma patient. Immediate initiation of prophylaxis is crucial in the absence of traumatic brain injury, spinal cord injury, or solid organ injury. In the case of creatinine clearance ranging from 30 to 60 ml/min, age greater than 65, weight less than 50 kg, or in the presence of pregnancy, it is recommended to administer enoxaparin at a dosage of 30 mg per day. If creatinine clearance is >30 ml/min, if there are no other criteria, and if body mass index is <30, enoxaparin should be started at 40 mg/day. If the

	Point
Underlying Conditions	
Obesity	2
Malignancy	2
Abnormal coagulation	2
History of VTE	3
Iatrogenic Factors	
Femoral vein line	2
Transfusion >4 units	2
Operation >2 hours	2
Major vein repair	3
Factors Associated with Injury	
Chest Abbreviated Injury Scale >2	2
Abdomen Abbreviated Injury Scale >2	2
Head Abbreviated Injury Scale >2	2
Spinal fractures	3
Glasgow coma score < 8	3
Serious lower extremity fracture	4
Pelvic fracture	4
Spinal cord injury	4
Age	
40–59	2
60–74	3
≥75	4

Table 6.
Risk assessment profile.

body mass index is >30, enoxaparin should be started at 0.5 mg/kg/day. If creatinine clearance is <30 ml/min and body mass index is <30, unfractional heparin 5000 IU should be administered every 8 hours. If body mass index is >30, unfractional heparin 7500 IU is recommended to be administered every 8 hours. The timing of prophylaxis in patients with traumatic brain injury should be determined by consulting the Modified Norwood Criteria. Enoxaparin 30 mg/day is recommended for VTE prophylaxis in eligible patients. In cases of spinal fracture or spinal cord injuries, prophylaxis should be initiated within 48 hours, and enoxaparin 30 mg per day should be administered. In cases of solid organ injuries without evidence of bleeding, VTE prophylaxis should commence within the first 48 hours, utilizing a daily dose of enoxaparin at 30 mg. However, if there is evidence of bleeding, chemoprophylaxis should not be applied; mechanical prophylaxis methods should be used [41].

4.4 Pregnant women

VTE can occur in about 1–2 out of every 1000 pregnant women [42–44]. The risk of VTE in pregnant women begins with the first trimester, the risk increases as the week of pregnancy increases, and the first postpartum period is the time when the risk is highest. When comparing pregnant and non-pregnant populations of the same age, a 15–35-fold increase in VTE risk was observed in pregnant women [45]. This risk is estimated to increase approximately 85 times during the first six weeks postpartum [46, 47]. As a result, seen during pregnancy, half of the PTE cases and one-third of the DVT cases occur after birth. This condition emphasizes that in the first postnatal period, the risk of developing VTE is highest. This risk begins to decrease from the 6th week after birth and returns to the initial risk by the 12th week [48]. VTE occurring during pregnancy and puerperium represents approximately 14% of maternal deaths in developed countries [49]. Previous history of VTE is considered the most critical risk factor in pregnant patients. For this reason, international guidelines recommend thromboprophylaxis for six weeks postpartum in pregnant women with a history of VTE [45, 50, 51]. Both prenatal and postpartum thromboprophylaxis are recommended for women with a history of unprovoked, pregnancy- or hormone replacement therapy-associated VTE. If antepartum thromboprophylaxis is indicated, LMWH should be started as soon as possible after pregnancy is confirmed. Only postpartum prophylaxis for six weeks is recommended for those who have had a single previous VTE due to a significant transient non-hormonal risk factor (e.g., trauma, surgery, immobilization) and those who have experienced VTE due to hormonal therapy [50]. Data on the use of antithrombotic therapy in women with thrombophilia and no history of VTE are limited. For this reason, the guidelines present different approaches to VTE prophylaxis in asymptomatic thrombophilia patients. Perhaps the most reasonable approach would be to evaluate general VTE risk factors in addition to the patient's asymptomatic thrombophilia and decide on VTE prophylaxis accordingly. Thromboprophylaxis is strongly recommended for high-risk thrombophilia patients with a positive family history of VTE during pregnancy. However, if there is no family history and the patient has low-risk thrombophilia, antepartum thromboprophylaxis is not recommended. Thromboprophylaxis is recommended for high-risk thrombophilia patients, even if there is no family history in the postpartum period [42, 52].

4.5 Hospitalized medical patients

Patients who are hospitalized and under medical supervision face a significant risk of VTE due to their immobility and underlying risk factors. Studies show that 42% of this patient group is at medium-high risk for VTE [53]. At the same time, VTE may develop in this patient group at a rate of 10–20% during hospitalization [10]. An autopsy study demonstrates that VTE contributes to approximately 10% of hospitalized patient deaths. Many of these patients were not diagnosed with VTE before they died [54]. As a result, VTE diagnosis may be delayed in these patient groups. It is essential to carefully evaluate this patient group's risk factors and VTE prophylaxis. It is also essential to evaluate the risk of bleeding in this patient group. Prophylaxis with enoxaparin 40 mg/day should be administered to appropriate patients. Mechanical prophylaxis may be considered in patients with a high risk of bleeding [55]. Studies recommended using the Padua risk score to assess the risk of VTE and initiate prophylaxis in high-risk patients [56, 57]. If the Padua risk score is four or above and there are no contraindications to thromboprophylaxis, VTE prophylaxis should be administered [58]. Details regarding the Padua risk score are given in **Table 7**.

DOI: http://dx.doi.org/10.5772/intechopen.1007194

Risk factor	Point
Age > 70	1
Arthritis/Active infection	1
Decreased mobility	3
Heart/Lung Failure	1
Body mass index >30	1
Active cancer	3
Ischemic stroke/myocardial infarction	1
Post thromboembolic event	3
Trauma/surgery within the last month	2
Thrombophilia	3
Hormone replacement therapy	1

Table 7.
Padua risk score.

5. Conclusion

DVT and VTE can cause severe morbidity and mortality. Knowing to whom and when to apply VTE prophylaxis, especially in specific patient groups, can significantly reduce preventable morbidity and mortality. Additionally, it is crucial to know the drugs used in VTE prophylaxis and their doses. Evaluating the risk of bleeding along with risk factors also provides clinical benefits. Mechanical prophylaxis can be used as an alternative to chemoprophylaxis in patients with severe bleeding risk for whom chemoprophylaxis cannot be administered.

Acknowledgements

The author(s) received no financial support for this chapter's research, authorship, and publication.

Conflict of interest

The authors declare no conflict of interest.

Author details

Sidar Şiyar Aydın* and Oğuzhan Birdal
Department of Cardiology, Faculty of Medicine, Ataturk University, Erzurum, Turkey

*Address all correspondence to: s.siyaraydin@gmail.com

References

[1] Cohen AT, Agnelli G, Anderson FA, et al. Venous thromboembolism (VTE) in Europe: The number of VTE events and associated morbidity and mortality. Thrombosis and Haemostasis. 2007;**98**(4):756-764

[2] Clagett GP, Anderson FA Jr, Geerts W, et al. Prevention of venous thromboembolism. Chest. 1998;**114**(5 Suppl):531S-560S. DOI: 10.1378/chest.114.5_supplement.531s

[3] Heit JA, Spencer FA, White RH. The epidemiology of venous thromboembolism. Journal of Thrombosis and Thrombolysis. 2016;**41**(1):3-14. DOI: 10.1007/s11239-015-1311-6

[4] Bell EJ, Lutsey PL, Basu S, et al. Lifetime risk of venous thromboembolism in two cohort studies. The American Journal of Medicine. 2016;**129**(3):339 e19-339 e26. DOI: 10.1016/j.amjmed.2015.10.014

[5] Roach RE, Cannegieter SC, Lijfering WM. Differential risks in men and women for first and recurrent venous thrombosis: The role of genes and environment. Journal of Thrombosis and Haemostasis. 2014;**12**(10):1593-1600. DOI: 10.1111/jth.12678

[6] Dentali F, Ageno W, Rancan E, et al. Seasonal and monthly variability in the incidence of venous thromboembolism. A systematic review and a meta-analysis of the literature. Thrombosis and Haemostasis. 2011;**106**(3):439-447. DOI: 10.1160/TH11-02-0116

[7] Braithwaite I, Healy B, Cameron L, Weatherall M, Beasley R. Venous thromboembolism risk associated with protracted work- and computer-related seated immobility: A case-control study. JRSM Open. 2016;7(8):2054270416632670. DOI: 10.1177/2054270416632670

[8] Franchini M, Mannucci PM. ABO blood group and thrombotic vascular disease. Thrombosis and Haemostasis. 2014;**112**(6):1103-1109. DOI: 10.1160/TH14-05-0457

[9] Olaf M, Cooney R. Deep venous thrombosis. Emergency Medicine Clinics of North America. 2017;**35**(4):743-770. DOI: 10.1016/j.emc.2017.06.003

[10] Cohen AT, Tapson VF, Bergmann JF, et al. Venous thromboembolism risk and prophylaxis in the acute hospital care setting (ENDORSE study): A multinational cross-sectional study. Lancet. 2008;**371**(9610):387-394. DOI: 10.1016/S0140-6736(08)60202-0

[11] Kearon C, Kahn SR, Agnelli G, Goldhaber S, Raskob GE, Comerota AJ. Antithrombotic therapy for venous thromboembolic disease: American College of Chest Physicians Evidence-Based Clinical Practice Guidelines (8th edition). Chest. 2008;**133**(6 Suppl):454S-545S. DOI: 10.1378/chest.08-0658

[12] Spencer FA, Emery C, Lessard D, et al. The Worcester venous thromboembolism study: A population-based study of the clinical epidemiology of venous thromboembolism. Journal of General Internal Medicine. 2006;**21**(7):722-727. DOI: 10.1111/j.1525-1497.2006.00458.x

[13] Bahl V, Hu HM, Henke PK, Wakefield TW, Campbell DA Jr, Caprini JA. A validation study of a retrospective venous thromboembolism risk scoring method. Annals of Surgery. 2010;**251**(2):344-350. DOI: 10.1097/SLA.0b013e3181b7fca6

[14] Schulman S, Kearon C, Kakkar AK, et al. Dabigatran versus warfarin in the treatment of acute venous thromboembolism. The New England Journal of Medicine. 2009;**361**(24):2342-2352. DOI: 10.1056/NEJMoa0906598

[15] Pastori D, Cormaci VM, Marucci S, et al. A comprehensive review of risk factors for venous thromboembolism: From epidemiology to pathophysiology. International Journal of Molecular Sciences. 2023;**24**(4):3169. DOI: 10.3390/ijms24043169

[16] Khorana AA, Dalal MR, Lin J, Connolly GC. Health care costs associated with venous thromboembolism in selected high-risk ambulatory patients with solid tumors undergoing chemotherapy in the United States. ClinicoEconomics and Outcomes Research. 2013;**5**:101-108. DOI: 10.2147/CEOR.S39964

[17] Khorana AA, Dalal M, Lin J, Connolly GC. Incidence and predictors of venous thromboembolism (VTE) among ambulatory high-risk cancer patients undergoing chemotherapy in the United States. Cancer. 2013;**119**(3):648-655. DOI: 10.1002/cncr.27772

[18] Farge D, Frere C, Connors JM, et al. 2022 international clinical practice guidelines for the treatment and prophylaxis of venous thromboembolism in patients with cancer, including patients with COVID-19. The Lancet Oncology. 2022;**23**(7):e334-e347. DOI: 10.1016/S1470-2045(22)00160-7

[19] Lyman GH, Carrier M, Ay C, et al. American Society of Hematology 2021 guidelines for management of venous thromboembolism: Prevention and treatment in patients with cancer. Blood Advances. 2021;**5**(4):927-974. DOI: 10.1182/bloodadvances.2020003442

[20] Munoz Martin AJ, Ortega I, Font C, et al. Multivariable clinical-genetic risk model for predicting venous thromboembolic events in patients with cancer. British Journal of Cancer. 2018;**118**(8):1056-1061. DOI: 10.1038/s41416-018-0027-8

[21] Munoz A, Ay C, Grilz E, et al. A clinical-genetic risk score for predicting cancer-associated venous thromboembolism: A development and validation study involving two independent prospective cohorts. Journal of Clinical Oncology. 2023;**41**(16):2911-2925. DOI: 10.1200/JCO.22.00255

[22] Streiff MB, Bockenstedt PL, Cataland SR, et al. Venous thromboembolic disease. Journal of the National Comprehensive Cancer Network. 2013;**11**(11):1402-1429. DOI: 10.6004/jnccn.2013.0163

[23] Caprini JA. Thrombosis risk assessment as a guide to quality patient care. Disease Month. 2005;**51**(2-3):70-78. DOI: 10.1016/j.disamonth.2005.02.003

[24] Bartlett MA, Mauck KF, Stephenson CR, Ganesh R, Daniels PR. Perioperative venous thromboembolism prophylaxis. Mayo Clinic Proceedings. 2020;**95**(12):2775-2798. DOI: 10.1016/j.mayocp.2020.06.015

[25] Pannucci CJ, Bailey SH, Dreszer G, et al. Validation of the Caprini risk assessment model in plastic and reconstructive surgery patients. Journal of the American College of Surgeons. 2011;**212**(1):105-112. DOI: 10.1016/j.jamcollsurg.2010.08.018

[26] Stroud W, Whitworth JM, Miklic M, et al. Validation of a venous thromboembolism risk assessment model in gynecologic oncology. Gynecologic Oncology. 2014;**134**(1):160-163. DOI: 10.1016/j.ygyno.2014.04.051

[27] Venclauskas L, Llau JV, Jenny JY, Kjaersgaard-Andersen P, Jans O, Force EVGT. European guidelines on perioperative venous thromboembolism prophylaxis: Day surgery and fast-track surgery. European Journal of Anaesthesiology. 2018;**35**(2):134-138. DOI: 10.1097/EJA.0000000000000706

[28] Cassidy MR, Rosenkranz P, McAneny D. Reducing postoperative venous thromboembolism complications with a standardized risk-stratified prophylaxis protocol and mobilization program. Journal of the American College of Surgeons. 2014;**218**(6):1095-1104. DOI: 10.1016/j.jamcollsurg.2013.12.061

[29] Pannucci CJ, Barta RJ, Portschy PR, et al. Assessment of postoperative venous thromboembolism risk in plastic surgery patients using the 2005 and 2010 Caprini risk score. Plastic and Reconstructive Surgery. 2012;**130**(2):343-353. DOI: 10.1097/PRS.0b013e3182589e49

[30] Jenny JY, Pabinger I, Samama CM, Force EVGT. European guidelines on perioperative venous thromboembolism prophylaxis: Aspirin. European Journal of Anaesthesiology. 2018;**35**(2):123-129. DOI: 10.1097/EJA.0000000000000728

[31] Falck-Ytter Y, Francis CW, Johanson NA, et al. Prevention of VTE in orthopedic surgery patients: Antithrombotic therapy and prevention of thrombosis, 9th ed—American College of Chest Physicians Evidence-Based Clinical Practice Guidelines. Chest. 2012;**141**(2 Suppl):e278S-e325S. DOI: 10.1378/chest.11-2404

[32] Carrier M, Altman AD, Blais N, et al. Extended thromboprophylaxis with low-molecular weight heparin (LMWH) following abdominopelvic cancer surgery. American Journal of Surgery. 2019;**218**(3):537-550. DOI: 10.1016/j.amjsurg.2018.11.046

[33] Gould MK, Garcia DA, Wren SM, et al. Prevention of VTE in nonorthopedic surgical patients: Antithrombotic therapy and prevention of thrombosis, 9th ed—American College of Chest Physicians Evidence-Based Clinical Practice Guidelines. Chest. 2012;**141**(2 Suppl):e227S-e277S. DOI: 10.1378/chest.11-2297

[34] Dong K, Song Y, Li X, et al. Pentasaccharides for the prevention of venous thromboembolism. Cochrane Database of Systematic Reviews. 2016;**10**(10):CD005134. DOI: 10.1002/14651858.CD005134.pub3

[35] Smythe MA, Priziola J, Dobesh PP, Wirth D, Cuker A, Wittkowsky AK. Guidance for the practical management of the heparin anticoagulants in the treatment of venous thromboembolism. Journal of Thrombosis and Thrombolysis. 2016;**41**(1):165-186. DOI: 10.1007/s11239-015-1315-2

[36] Bendinelli C, Balogh Z. Postinjury thromboprophylaxis. Current Opinion in Critical Care. 2008;**14**(6):673-678. DOI: 10.1097/MCC.0b013e3283196538

[37] Dunbar NM, Chandler WL. Thrombin generation in trauma paticnts. Transfusion. 2009;**49**(12):2652-2660. DOI: 10.1111/j.1537-2995.2009.02335.x

[38] Toker S, Hak DJ, Morgan SJ. Deep vein thrombosis prophylaxis in trauma patients. Thrombosis. 2011;**2011**:505373. DOI: 10.1155/2011/505373

[39] Greenfield LJ, Proctor MC, Rodriguez JL, Luchette FA, Cipolle MD, Cho J. Posttrauma thromboembolism prophylaxis. The Journal of Trauma. 1997;**42**(1):100-103. DOI: 10.1097/00005373-199701000-00017

[40] Gearhart MM, Luchette FA, Proctor MC, et al. The risk assessment

profile score identifies trauma patients at risk for deep vein thrombosis. Surgery. 2000;**128**(4):631-640. DOI: 10.1067/msy.2000.108224

[41] Yorkgitis BK, Berndtson AE, Cross A, et al. American Association for the Surgery of Trauma/American College of Surgeons-Committee on trauma clinical protocol for inpatient venous thromboembolism prophylaxis after trauma. Journal of Trauma and Acute Care Surgery. 2022;**92**(3):597-604. DOI: 10.1097/TA.0000000000003475

[42] Hart C, Bauersachs R, Scholz U, et al. Prevention of venous thromboembolism during pregnancy and the puerperium with a special focus on women with hereditary thrombophilia or prior VTE-position paper of the working group in women's health of the society of thrombosis and haemostasis (GTH). Hämostaseologie. 2020;**40**(5):572-590. DOI: 10.1055/a-1132-0750

[43] Parunov LA, Soshitova NP, Ovanesov MV, Panteleev MA, Serebriyskiy II. Epidemiology of venous thromboembolism (VTE) associated with pregnancy. Birth Defects Research. Part C, Embryo Today. 2015;**105**(3):167-184. DOI: 10.1002/bdrc.21105

[44] Kourlaba G, Relakis J, Kontodimas S, Holm MV, Maniadakis N. A systematic review and meta-analysis of the epidemiology and burden of venous thromboembolism among pregnant women. International Journal of Gynaecology and Obstetrics. 2016;**132**(1):4-10. DOI: 10.1016/j.ijgo.2015.06.054

[45] Bates SM, Middeldorp S, Rodger M, James AH, Greer I. Guidance for the treatment and prevention of obstetric-associated venous thromboembolism. Journal of Thrombosis and Thrombolysis. 2016;**41**(1):92-128. DOI: 10.1007/s11239-015-1309-0

[46] Jackson E, Curtis KM, Gaffield ME. Risk of venous thromboembolism during the postpartum period: A systematic review. Obstetrics and Gynecology. 2011;**117**(3):691-703. DOI: 10.1097/AOG.0b013e31820ce2db

[47] Sultan AA, West J, Tata LJ, Fleming KM, Nelson-Piercy C, Grainge MJ. Risk of first venous thromboembolism in and around pregnancy: A population-based cohort study. British Journal of Haematology. 2012;**156**(3):366-373. DOI: 10.1111/j.1365-2141.2011.08956.x

[48] Kamel H, Navi BB, Sriram N, Hovsepian DA, Devereux RB, Elkind MS. Risk of a thrombotic event after the 6-week postpartum period. The New England Journal of Medicine. 2014;**370**(14):1307-1315. DOI: 10.1056/NEJMoa1311485

[49] Abbasi N, Balayla J, Laporta DP, Kezouh A, Abenhaim HA. Trends, risk factors and mortality among women with venous thromboembolism during labour and delivery: A population-based study of 8 million births. Archives of Gynecology and Obstetrics. 2014;**289**(2):275-284. DOI: 10.1007/s00404-013-2923-8

[50] Bates SM, Greer IA, Middeldorp S, Veenstra DL, Prabulos AM, Vandvik PO. VTE, thrombophilia, antithrombotic therapy, and pregnancy: Antithrombotic therapy and prevention of thrombosis, 9th ed—American College of Chest Physicians Evidence-Based Clinical Practice Guidelines. Chest. 2012;**141**(2 Suppl):e691S-e736S. DOI: 10.1378/chest.11-2300

[51] Chan WS, Rey E, Kent NE, et al. Venous thromboembolism and antithrombotic therapy in pregnancy. Journal of Obstetrics and Gynaecology Canada. 2014;**36**(6):527-553. DOI: 10.1016/s1701-2163(15)30569-7

[52] Bistervels IM, Scheres LJJ, Hamulyak EN, Middeldorp S. Sex matters: Practice 5P's when treating young women with venous thromboembolism. Journal of Thrombosis and Haemostasis. 2019;**17**(9):1417-1429. DOI: 10.1111/jth.14549

[53] Dobromirski M, Cohen AT. How I manage venous thromboembolism risk in hospitalized medical patients. Blood. 2012;**120**(8):1562-1569. DOI: 10.1182/blood-2012-03-378901

[54] Lindblad B, Sternby NH, Bergqvist D. Incidence of venous thromboembolism verified by necropsy over 30 years. BMJ. 1991;**302**(6778):709-711. DOI: 10.1136/bmj.302.6778.709

[55] Mahlab-Guri K, Otman MS, Replianski N, Rosenberg-Bezalel S, Rabinovich I, Sthoeger Z. Venous thromboembolism prophylaxis in patients hospitalized in medical wards: A real life experience. Medicine (Baltimore). 2020;**99**(7):e19127. DOI: 10.1097/MD.0000000000019127

[56] Chandra D, Dabhi K, Lester W. Are we assessing venous thromboembolism (VTE) risk appropriately for hospitalised medical patients? The national VTE risk assessment tool versus Padua prediction score. British Journal of Haematology. 2020;**189**(1):e16-e18. DOI: 10.1111/bjh.16411

[57] Zhou C, Guang Y, Luo Y, et al. Superior predictive value of D-dimer to the Padua prediction score for venous thromboembolism in inpatients with AECOPD: A multicenter cohort study. International Journal of Chronic Obstructive Pulmonary Disease. 2022;**17**:2711-2722. DOI: 10.2147/COPD.S380418

[58] Barbar S, Noventa F, Rossetto V, et al. A risk assessment model for the identification of hospitalized medical patients at risk for venous thromboembolism: The Padua prediction score. Journal of Thrombosis and Haemostasis. 2010;**8**(11):2450-2457. DOI: 10.1111/j.1538-7836.2010.04044.x

Chapter 3

Perspective Chapter: Deep Vein Thrombosis Prevention in Patients with Solid Organ Injuries

Gary J. Curcio

Abstract

Deep Vein Thrombosis can be a very serious complication in the traumatically injuries patient. Those with solid organ injuries present with some unique issues as well. Failure of non-operative or even operative management resulting on going or rebleeding are the most serious issue these patients face. Timing of Deep vein thrombosis, DVT, prophylaxis has traditionally been a topic of discussion in patients with solid organ injuries. In the medical literature there is an increasing amount of information to help assist with this issue. Most notably in the traumatically injuries patient with a traumatic brain injury. The literature is not quit as abundant for traumatically injured patients with solid organ injuries. This chapter will look at some of the literature and practice guidelines to help the reader make the best determination on timing of deep vein thrombosis prophylaxis.

Keywords: deep vein thrombosis, deep vein thrombosis prophylaxis, chemical prophylaxis, mechanical prophylaxis, solid organ, endovascular, solid organ injury grading, heparin induced thrombocytopenia

1. Introduction

Patients with traumatic injuries can be complex and have several competing issues that need to be address to assure the best outcome. These can range from ambulation, to treatment for their traumatic injuries, to restarting home medication. This can be compounded by pre-existing conditions that may require contraindicating therapies based on a new injury pattern. It is not unusual for a patient to be on an anticoagulant or antiplatelet with an acute injury that has caused hemorrhaging. To compound these issues there will be consultants recommending conflicting therapies based on the patient pre-existing conditions and/or their acute injuries.

Traumatically injured patient are at the highest risk of developing deep vein thrombosis, (DVT), and subsequent complications such as pulmonary embolisms. DVT are potentially preventable in traumatically injuries patients. Several algorithms have been developed to prevent DVT as well as the complication that can occur with

DVT [1, 2]. The Therapies range from mechanical prophylaxis, chemical prophylaxis or alternative means. Chemical prophylaxis is the mainstay of therapy. There is a fear from providers to initiate chemical DVT therapying in a timely fashion. This fear is because of the chance of increased or continued hemorrhage. This fear real as it can lead to poor outcomes in the event of ongoing or recurrent hemorrhage. The fear of hemorrhage and lack of reversal agents also compounds this problem.

Many subspecialists have their own though and practices based on past experiences and are not necessarily based on the best available literature on the topic. Less experienced provider can also delay appropriate DVT therapy leading to unnecessary complications. This delay in appropriate DVT prevention can lead to increased risk of morbidity and mortality in patients. Trauma patient have been identified as high risk for DVT and this delay can have catastrophic effects on the patient recovery. The delay can lead to increased length of stay in the hospital, ventilation days, intensive care days and morbidity and mortality [3].

All this can become over whelming very quickly. Of late, there has been a lot of attention in the area of Traumatic Brain Injury and DVT prevention. Several studies and guidelines have been developed over the years to help guide this problem [1, 4, 5]. There is much less literature on the subject of deep vein thrombosis prevention and solid organ injuries.

This chapter with focus on solid organ injuries. The topics will range from identifying the extent of the injuries. We will use the known grading system to standardize the grades assigned. What is the risk of bleeding with each grade of injury? The different types of DVT prophylaxis are available with each grade of injury. Does the grade of injury relate to the risk of bleeding with DVT prophylaxis? Each organ will be broken down using the above mentioned criteria.

The goal of this chapter is to identify the patient with a solid organ injury from a traumatic event. The grading system used to identify the injury and with each grade the risk of bleeding. To identify the appropriate DVT and the timing of the initiation of the therapy. How to monitor these patients and the setting this monitoring should be conducted such as floor verse intensive care setting. How long they should be monitored in the critical care setting. What monitoring should be utilized such as cardiac monitoring, laboratory studies vital statistics, and specialized studies etc.

When DVT therapy is initiated what is the best form of therapy to be used; chemical, mechanical or endovascular procedures. The duration of the therapy in the hospital setting and the outpatient and rehab or skilled nursing setting.

The options for DVT prophylaxis in patients that are at low and high risk of bleeding vary. Is the timing of initiation of DVT prophylaxis based on the organ grade or other factors? The setting this should be done in and what intervention can be used if bleeding occurs. Finally, to summarize the recommendation available to guide therapy.

2. Types of deep vein thrombosis therapy

There are multiple ways to prevent DVT. Whether they are mechanical, chemical or endovascular, they have role in the prevention of DVT. Depending on the patient's unique condition including; injuries, preexisting medical condition and medication one option may be superior to another. This will help guide which for option should be utilized.

2.1 Mechanical

Sequential Compression Devices utilized intermittent compression on the extremities to mimic the pumping action of the lower extremity muscle contraction to facilitate blood flow from the extremity to the heart. Studies as far back at the 2002 shows that when used properly they are non-inferior to chemical prophylaxis. Properly is defined at sequential compression devices applied to the lower extremities for 22 of 24 hours [2, 4].

2.2 Chemical

Chemical prophylaxis can be accomplished by utilizing low dose unfractionated heparin or low molecular weight heparins. In the trauma patient low dose molecular heparin are preferred, [5, 6]. Several guidelines have been established to reinforce this recommendation [1, 2, 7].

2.3 Endovascular procedures

These endovascular procedures are done by several medical specialties, (Vascular surgery, General Surgery, Interventional Radiology). This is accomplished by placing an Inferior Vena Cava Filter. These are placed in the descending inferior vena cava below the renal veins. Many of these filters are designed to be retrieved and should be removed once they are no longer needed. These filters should be removed once the patient's hemoglobin has stabilized and they have tolerated DVT prophylaxis by chemical means without a further drop in the hemoglobin concentration. This can limit and morbidity related to the devices [7].

3. Grading of solid organ injuries

The American Association for the Surgery of Trauma, AAST, has developed a grading system for traumatically injured systems of the body [8]. These include solid organ injuries as well. The solid organs of the abdominal cavity are; liver, spleen, kidney, adrenal, pancreas, and ovaries. The testis and scrotum and added to the group even though they are technically not in the abdominal cavity.

The grading system applies a number, 1 through 5, to describe the extent of injures. As the number gets higher, the extent of damage is more severe. This grading system is based on radiology finding from a computer tomography scan. This grading system has is acceptance and is a common nomenclature when describing solid organ injuries. Anatomic Based injury Severity Score, AIS, is also referenced with regards to solid organ injuries. As with the AAST solid organ grading system, there greater the injury the higher the score [3].

3.1 Liver injuries

Liver injuries are the most common solid organ injury in the abdominal cavity. They typically are non-operative in the lower grades and angiography has taken a larger role in their management. Surgical repair of liver injuries is reserved for unstable patients or in patients that non operative management failed. Liver injuries are one of the more common solid organs injured by the nature of their relative size to the other intra-abdominal solid organs. Other associated injuries with liver trauma are rib and diaphragm injuries. The liver injuries are graded per the AAST grading system. The injuries with lower severity are grade 1–3. These tend to be treated non operatively. Liver injuries are amendable to endovascular techniques to stop hemorrhaging. Mid to higher grade injuries in hemodynamically stable patients are best suited for endovascular therapies. Higher grade injuries, (4–5), in unstable patients have higher rates of conservative management failure requiring operative management [3, 9, 10].

3.2 Splenic injuries

Splenic injuries occur with primarily blunt abdominal trauma but can occur in penetrating trauma as well. Often there are associate injuries similar to liver injuries. The splenic injuries are also associated with rib fractures and diaphragmatic injuries. As with Liver injuries, lower grade injuries are typically treated in a nonoperative fashion and high grade with angioembolization. Surgical removal or repair of splenic injuries are reserved for unstable patients or those that have failed non operative management similar to liver injuries. Similar to liver injuries, lower grade splenic injuries tended to be treated non operatively. Endovascular approaches to control hemorrhage from the spleen are very effective in hemodynamically stable patients. Unlike liver injuries higher grade splenic injuries are managed with splenectomy where liver injuries are managed surgically with operative repair [3, 11].

3.3 Kidney injuries

Kidney injuries are seen in blunt and penetrating trauma. Even though the kidneys are located in the retroperitoneum. The kidneys are classified as intraabdominal solid organ. Typically, kidney injures and not surgically explored unless there are other reasons to go to the operating room with the patient. Similar to liver and splenic injuries, kidney injuries, can be controlled with various endovascular techniques. Hematuria, abdominal hematomas and uromas are common finding in higher grade injuries and should be looked for [3, 9].

3.4 Ovarian injuries

Ovarian injuries are not as common as other solid intraabdominal organ injuries. They are unique in that they are a bilateral true intraabdominal organ and with bilateral injuries their grade is upgraded. For example, a grade one ovarian contusion that is bilateral becomes a grade three injury [3, 12].

3.5 Pancreas injuries

Pancreatic injuries are seldomly seen in isolation just by the nature of their location in the abdominal cavity. These injuries are typically paired with duodenal injuries when the proximal pancreas is involved. Distal injuries are commonly associated with splenic injuries. Miss pancreatic injuries can lead to high morbidity and mortality. Pancreatic injuries are by their location very difficult to manage. The mainstay of surgical management is initially by wide drainage. Magnetic Resonance Cholangio

Pancreatography and Endoscopic Cholangiopancreatography are typically ancillary procedures used to assist with the grading of pancreatic injuries [3, 13].

3.6 Testes and scrotum injuries

These structures are not typically seen in the abdominal cavity but the origin of the testes is in the abdominal cavity as a fetus. They can be located in the abdominal cavity when the testes is undescended. Similar to ovarian injuries, lower grade Testicular injuries result in a higher grade [3, 11].

4. Timing of deep vein thrombosis prophylaxis

The timing of DVT prophylaxis is essential in the trauma patient with solid organ injury. These patients are a higher risk of DVT and subsequent complication such as pulmonary embolism.

The appropriate time of chemical prophylaxis is not a straight forward topic. The risk of hemorrhage and nonoperative management as well as the risk of DVT need to be taken into consideration. The literature supports early deep vein thrombosis by chemical means which is defined as starting prophylaxis in less than 48 hours, ideally within 12–24 hours of injury. There is a small risk of failure with nonoperative management of solid organ injuries. Increased failure rates are defined as the present of DVT and increased transfusion rates. When early prophylaxis was initiated, mortality was improved. The failure rate in early chemical prophylaxis is low [14].

Stable hemoglobin concentration can be used to assist with guiding early chemical prophylaxis for solid organ injuries. After a stable hemoglobin concentration for 12–24 hours in solid organ injuries, chemical prophylaxis can be initiated. Stable hemoglobin concentration at 12–24 hours can be used as a maker to predict if the patient will fail non operative management [6].

The grade of solid organ injury has less of an effect on the initiation of DVT prevention and more on the type of prophylaxis utilized. The grade of the organ injury has not been linked to need for delays in early DVT prophylaxis. Although with higher grade of injuries hemoglobin concentration may take longer to stabilize. This may require alternative means of prophylaxis such and Inferior Vena Cava Filters and Sequential Compression Devices in place of chemical prophylaxis. Higher grade injuries should be admitted to a monitored bed or Intensive Care Unit depending on the hospital's resources. Serial laboratory studies should be obtained to trend the hemoglobin concentration and establish when it has become stable. Lower grade injuries can be admitted to a step down unit. Serial laboratory studies and vital statistic should be monitored. High grade injuries may delay the initiation of chemical prophylaxis but should not delay starting appropriate DVT prophylaxis. The overall goal should still be to initiate chemical prophylaxis as soon as the hemoglobin concentration is stable where other means of prophylaxis have been started already.

Delays in starting DVT prophylaxis correlates with a high rate of developing DVT in trauma patients. The trauma patient has long been identified as a high risk group for DVT. The increase in morbidity and mortality is the greatest concern. The need for early, safe prophylaxis has been a topic in the medical literature. The results are showing reduction in complication when early DVT prophylaxis with early, <24 hours compared to late, > 24 hours for the initiation of therapy [1].

5. Deep vein thrombosis chemical prophylaxis

Chemical DVT prophylaxis is the preferred therapy. In trauma patients low molecular weight heparins are the preferred therapy. Low molecular weight heparin and was first approved for medical use in 1993 and is derived from heparin. It has a quick onset of action; 2 hours and it effects last for up to 12 hours. It is an indirect anticoagulant that binds and potentiates antithrombin III (serine protease inhibitor) through a specific pentasaccharide sequence to form a complex that irreversibly inactivates factor Xa [15]. The preferred dose is a weigh based dose, (0.5 mg/kg), (6,11). Contraindication to low molecular weight heparin would primarily be in a patient with acute renal failure or chronic renal insufficiency with a creatine about 2.0 mg/dl.

In patient's where low molecular weight heparin is contraindicated then unfractionated heparin would be the primary choice. Unfractionated heparin is a sulfated. It produces its major anticoagulant effect by inactivating thrombin and activated factor X (factor Xa) through an antithrombin (AT)-dependent mechanism. Heparin binds to AT through a high-affinity pentasaccharide, which is present on about a third of heparin molecules [16]. A dose of 5000 unit administered 3 times per day is the preferred dose for DVT prophylaxis.

In the event that bleeding does occur there was several methods to address this. The initial steps should be to reverse the effects of the chemical prophylaxis used. For unfractionated heparin or low molecular heparin, Protamine, is the initial drug of choice for reversal. Other options, if there is an identified source of bleeding, wound be Interventional Radiologic procedures if available. Catheter based approaches to bleeding control have made advances in recent years. Finally, as a last option surgical intervention is an option.

There are circumstances where low molecular weight heparins and unfractionated heparins are contraindicated. The most notable would be heparin induced thrombocytopenia. In this condition the use of either medication will result in thrombocytopenia. The diagnosis is made when a reduction of the platelet count is <100,000 or a 50% drop in the absolute platelet value after initiation of one of these medications. This can result in an increased hemorrhage risk in these patients. If the patient develops a thrombocytosis or relative drop in platelet count by 50% then Heparin Inducted Thrombocytopenia should be considered.

Heparin inducted thrombocytopenia, (HIT) has two main categories. The first, known as HIT-1 results on a drop the platelet count as previously stated. It is a nonimmune mediated reaction to these two medications typically used for DVT prophylaxis. The second being HIT-2, this is an autoimmune response. There is the formation of antibodies that activate platelets following the administration of low molecular weight and unfractionated heparins. This can result in not only venous but arterial thrombosis.

The therapy for HIT –1 is immediate discontinuation of low molecular weight and or unfractionated heparin and starting fondaparinox at the deep vein thrombosis prophylaxis dose of 0.5 mg subcutaneously daily. With HIT-2 administration of full dose Leperudin or Argatroban is necessary to treat the possible thrombotic effects of HIT-2 [17].

6. Alternative to chemical prophylaxis

In the event that the patient's hemoglobin is not stable, other non-chemical methods can be utilized for DVT prophylaxis. The most common and least invasive would be

Sequential Compression Devices. Contraindication to using Sequential Compression Devices would be; known extremity clots on the limb where the device is placed, open wound to the area the device is being applied, severe peripheral arterial occlusive disease of the extremity as well as compartment syndrome of the extremity.

The use of other medication such as antiplatelets and medication classified as direct oral anticoagulants are not used in DVT prevention presently. There is no real literature to support their use for prevention of DVT. Although, there is a growing body of evidence in the use for treatment of DVT or pulmonary embolism with direct oral anticoagulants [9]. At present the use of antiplatelet or direct oral anticoagulants should not be used for the primary prevention of deep vein thrombosis.

Sequential Compression Devices have been shown be very successful in preventing deep vein thrombosis and pulmonary embolisms when used properly. Unfortunately, there proper use has come into question. In some instances, they are used improperly in 80% of the patients followed [4]. When used properly, their use is associated with reduction in the deep vein thrombosis risk and with very low complication rates.

When Chemical prophylaxis cannot be instituted or if sequential compression devices cannot be used, then inferior vena cava filters are an option. This are an invasive procedure with risks associated with their placement and use. Current inferior vena cava filters are retrievable. That is, they are designed to be removed once they are no longer needed. Typical complication are bleeding at insertion site, deployment malfunctions, infection, blockage of the injury to the inferior vena cava, migration of the device and fracture of the device and injury to the inferior vena cava [8].

7. Conclusion

In Conclusion, DVT can lead to significant morbidity and mortality in trauma patients. The prevention is paramount in limiting the risk of complication related to DVT. The appropriate method of prevention and the timing of prevention are key to successful limitation of deep vein thrombosis. Traumatically injured patients are at high risk for DVT. Patient with solid organ injuries are not exempt from this risk. Proper DVT prophylaxis is crucial to preventing DVT and the complication that are associated with them. There are several options to prevent DVT in traumatically injured patient with solid organ injuries. Early DVT prophylaxis has been shown to be safe and reduces the morbidity and mortality in this patient population.

Author details

Gary J. Curcio
Morsani School of Medicine, University of South Florida, Tampa, Florida, USA

*Address all correspondence to: drgcurcio@gmail.com

References

[1] Ley, Eric J, Brown CVR, Moore Ernest E, Sava Jack A, Kimberly P, Ciesla David J, et al. Updated guidelines to reduce venous thromboembolism in trauma patients: A Western trauma association critical decisions algorithm. Journal of Trauma and Acute Care Surgery. 2020;**89**(5):971-981

[2] The EAST Practice Management Guidelines Work Group, Rogers FB, Cipolle MD, Velmahos G, Rozycki G, Luchette FA. Practice management guidelines for the prevention of venous thromboembolism in trauma patients. Trauma. 2002;**53**:142-164

[3] Rappold JF, Sheppard FR, Carmichael II SP, Cuschieri J, Ley E, Rangel E, et al. Venous thromboembolism prophylaxis in the trauma intensive care unit: An American association for the, surgery of trauma critical care committee clinical consensus document. Trauma Surgery & Acute Care Open. 2021;**6**(1):1-8

[4] Cornwell EE 3rd, Chang D, Velmahos G, Jindal A, Baker D, Phillips J, et al. Compliance with sequential compression device prophylaxis in at-risk trauma patients: A prospective analysis. The American Surgeon. 2002;**68**(5):470-473

[5] Steinke B, Geisel L, Hobbs B, Perry M, Birrer K, Liu X, et al. Venous thromboembolism prophylaxis in surgery and trauma patients. 24 Oct 2023:1-5 Available from: www.criticalcare.net

[6] Marturano MN, Khan AR, DeBlieux P, Wang H, Ross SW, Cunningham KW, et al. Timing of venous thromboembolism chemoprophylaxis using objective hemoglobin criteria in blunt solid organ injury. Injury. 2023;**54**(5):1356-1361

[7] Russo R, Gamble B, Bradley M, Van Gent M, Tadlock MD, How RA, et al. Prevention of Venous Thromboembolism, to Establish Guidance for Anti-Thrombotic Therapy for the Prevention of Deep Venous Thrombosis and Pulmonary Embolism and the Management of Inferior Vena Cava Filters Placed in Theater for Primary or Secondary Prophylaxis of Pulmonary Embolism. Joint Trauma System Clinical Practice Guidelines (JTS CPG). 2024

[8] Ahmed I, Majeed A, Powell R. Heparin induced thrombocytopenia: Diagnosis and management update. Postgraduate Medical Journal. 2007;**83**(983):575-582

[9] Beltzer C, Imach S, Wafaisaade A, Lefering R, Koible B, Langenbeck's Archives of Surgery. Atlas of Emergency Imaging Form Head to Toe. Springer Science and Business media LLC; 2022

[10] Lorenz J, Van Ha TG. Complications in interventional radiology. Seminars in Interventional Radiology. 2006;**23**(2):150-155

[11] The Egyptian Urological Guidelines on Lower Urinary Tract and Genitalia Trauma Chapter 8 pages VIII. 3.1-Definitions of Trauma, pages VIII. 3.2 Classification of Trauma, and pages VIII. 3.3 Urogenital Trauma

[12] Hill P, Suresh K. Chapter 8 Imaging of Genitourinary Trauma, Joanie Garett, jay Im, Akshya Guptsa. Springer Science and Business Meida LLC. US Military: Joint Trauma System Clinical practic Guidelines; 2023

[13] Waqas S, Ashraf MS, Khan MAM. Multidisciplinary management of high-grade pediatric liver injuries. European

Journal of Trauma Emergency Surgery. 2024;**50**:829-836

[14] Lamb T, Lenet T, Zahrai A, Shaw JR, McLarty R, Shorr R, et al. Timing of pharmacologic venous thromboembolism prophylaxis initiation for trauma patients with nonoperatively managed blunt abdominal solid organ injury: A systematic review and meta-analysis. World Journal of Emergency Surgery. 2022;**17**:19

[15] Jupalli A, Muhamad A. National Institute of Health. USA. 28 Aug 2023

[16] Hirsh J, Anand SS, Halperin J, Fuster V. Mechanism of action and pharmacology of unfractionated heparin. AHA/ASA Journals. 2001;21(7)

[17] Schreiber D, Brenner BE. Anticoagulation in deep venous thrombosis. USA: Medscape. 2020

Chapter 4

Venous Thromboembolism in Patients with Acute Brain Injury

Mostafa A. AL Turk

Abstract

Venous thromboembolism (VTE) represents a significant and unpredictable complication during any hospital stay. Patients with neurological injuries are at a particularly higher risk for such complications. Both prophylaxis and treatment of VTE in these patients present challenging and often controversial topics for intensivists and neurologists. The abundance of research and guidelines available for treating stroke and traumatic brain injury patients has facilitated the prevention and management of thromboembolisms in this subset of patients. On the other hand, patients with aneurysmal subarachnoid hemorrhage can be safely initiated on anticoagulation therapy once the bleeding vessel is secured. However, patients with spontaneous intraparenchymal hemorrhage have traditionally been overlooked in terms of VTE prophylaxis. Given the complexity and variability in clinical presentations, a tailored approach is essential. This involves balancing the risks of thromboembolism against the potential for exacerbating intracranial bleeding. Emerging evidence and evolving guidelines continue to shape best practices, aiming to optimize outcomes for these vulnerable patient populations.

Keywords: venous thromboembolism, unfractionated heparin, low molecular weight heparin, acute ischemic stroke, traumatic brain injury, spontaneous intraparenchymal bleed, aneurysmal subarachnoid hemorrhage

1. Introduction

Venous thromboembolism (VTE) represents a significant and often underappreciated complication in patients with neurological injuries, including traumatic brain injury (TBI), acute ischemic stroke, and intracranial hemorrhage. These conditions not only predispose patients to VTE due to prolonged immobility and endothelial injury but also present unique challenges in balancing the risks of thrombosis and hemorrhage.

In the neurocritical care setting, the management of VTE prophylaxis and treatment requires a nuanced approach that considers the delicate interplay between preventing thromboembolic events and minimizing the risk of exacerbating intracranial bleeding. The pathophysiology of VTE in these patients is multifaceted, involving factors such as venous stasis, hypercoagulability, and direct vascular injury.

IntechOpen

This chapter delves into the latest evidence-based strategies for VTE prophylaxis and treatment in patients with TBI, acute ischemic stroke, and intracranial hemorrhage. It explores the timing and selection of pharmacologic and mechanical prophylaxis, the role of individualized risk assessment, and the impact of emerging therapies. By integrating clinical guidelines with real-world practice insights, this chapter aims to provide a comprehensive framework for optimizing patient outcomes in this high-risk population.

2. VTE in patients with acute brain injury

2.1 Traumatic brain injury

VTE is a common hospital complication, affecting approximately six hundred thousand patients in the USA yearly [1, 2]. TBI patients appear to be particularly susceptible, with a VTE incidence of about 20% in patients receiving VTE prophylaxis, reaching up to 58% in some reports [3]. Patients with severe TBI often require aggressive intracranial pressure (ICP) reduction, achieved through the induction of barbiturate coma or the use of neuromuscular blockers. This explains the higher-than-usual VTE incidence [4]. Other patient-specific factors associated with VTE development include younger age, skipping one or more chemoprophylaxis doses, and the need for neurosurgical intervention [5].

Chemoprophylaxis is proven to be effective in reducing the incidence of VTE, without affecting mortality [6]. However, due to concerns about exacerbating existing intracranial hemorrhage, many clinicians prefer to defer chemoprophylaxis for as long as 72 hours after hospitalization. This practice is based on several published studies showing comparable outcomes and complications of anticoagulation in patients receiving chemoprophylaxis either early (within 72 hours) or late (more than 72 hours) after hospital admission [7, 8]. Unfortunately, VTE can develop as soon as a couple of hours after hospital admission, especially in critically ill patients admitted to the intensive care unit (ICU). In other words, patients in the early group might be developing VTE even before anticoagulation is initiated.

The use of anticoagulation in these patients has always been a topic of controversy. The Brain Trauma Foundation released its fourth edition of the guidelines for the management of TBI in 2017 [9]. This edition included a level III recommendation for the use of low molecular heparin (LMWH) or low-dose unfractionated heparin (UFH) along with mechanical prophylaxis for VTE prevention. However, due to insufficient evidence, it did not include any recommendations regarding the optimal agent, timing of initiation, or doses.

Some institutions prefer to start chemoprophylaxis after a 24 h stability head CT scan has been performed, while others prefer to wait for the 48 h mark. Level I trauma centers have been known to start VTE prophylaxis earlier than level II centers, without any significantly different clinical outcomes [1]. It might be smart to continue doing neurological checks every 1 h after initiating chemoprophylaxis.

Several recently published small cohorts have investigated the optimal agent for chemoprophylaxis in this subset of patients. LMWH consistently demonstrates superiority in terms of VTE prevention [10, 11], and it even shows reduced hemorrhagic complications [10]. The optimal dosing also remains uncertain. UFH doses can vary from 5000 IU twice to three times a day, and up to 7500 IU three times a day in obese patients, administered subcutaneously. Enoxaparin, the most widely used LMWH, can be administered as 40 mg subcutaneously once or twice a day. Notably, one cohort demonstrated stable clinical outcomes in TBI patients who received LMWH at a dose of 40 mg twice a day [12]. However, these studies are limited to cohorts, and future randomized trials are strongly warranted.

Vigorous neurological monitoring is warranted in TBI patients, especially in severe cases and during the first few days post-injury. Clinicians should be vigilant in recognizing any worsening neurological symptoms after initiating chemoprophylaxis and promptly order appropriate studies, typically an emergent head CT, to check for any new or worsening intracranial bleeding.

2.2 Acute ischemic stroke

Patients with acute ischemic stroke are inherently at higher risk of VTE compared to other hospitalized patients. They exhibit two of the three components of Virchow's triad. On one hand, hemiplegia significantly limits their mobility compared to other bedridden patients. On the other hand, having experienced a stroke renders them in a hypercoagulable state. This theory is supported by the rates of VTE in this patient subset, which reach 75% [13], in contrast to 10% among other patients [14].

2.2.1 Chemoprophylaxis in patients with acute ischemic stroke

Initiating VTE chemoprophylaxis is not straightforward. Canadian stroke guidelines recommend starting chemoprophylaxis, using LMWH or UFH, on the day of admission for all patients are deemed high risk for developing VTE (such as those who are dehydrated, have one or more paralyzed limbs, cannot move independently, or have suspected or active malignancy) and do not have any contraindications [15]. In contrast, the US guidelines state that there is no proven benefit of subcutaneous heparin for VTE prophylaxis in patients with acute ischemic stroke [16]. Although the US guidelines do not specifically comment on the timing of initiation, they emphasize that if initiated, there is no benefit of LMWH over UFH. Both sets of guidelines, however, recommend the use of intermittent compressive devices (ICP) to be started at admission for VTE prophylaxis. It is worth noting that while the Canadian stroke guidelines were revised in 2022, the US AHA/ASA stroke guidelines were last revised in 2019, which may explain the differences in recommendations.

Many patients receive either IV alteplase or undergo thrombectomy at the time of presentation, which increases the risk of hemorrhagic conversion of their acute ischemic stroke if they were started on anticoagulation too soon. Initiating chemoprophylaxis after administering IV alteplase better be done 24 h hours later, allowing the alteplase effect to wane [16]. Starting chemoprophylaxis after thrombectomy better also be done 24 h after the procedure in order to mitigate the increased risk of hemorrhagic conversion [16].

2.2.2 The optimal anticoagulant

Several recently published studies have investigated the optimal agent for VTE prophylaxis is patients with acute ischemic stroke. A large cohort found that LMWH was effective as UFH for VTE prevention and, surprisingly, had a protective effect in terms of hemorrhagic conversion [17].

This is contrary to the general belief that UFH is safer and caries less risk of hemorrhagic conversion compared to LWMH. Additionally, the fact that protamine sulfate can neutralize UFH to a greater extent than neutralizing LMWH [18, 19] have contributed its persistent adoption by many neurosurgeons and neurointensivists. A possible explanation for the protective effect of LMWH is that is has more antithrombin and less anticoagulant activity when compared to UFH [20, 21].

The size of the ischemic stroke also plays a significant role. Larger strokes are at higher risk of hemorrhagic conversion, and physicians need to weigh the risks versus benefits of starting chemoprophylaxis for these patients. Additionally, patients with large strokes are sometimes placed on a hemicraniectomy watch (to relieve the compression if the swelling gets more severe), thus chemoprophylaxis is usually deferred until this phase is over.

2.2.3 Chemoprophylaxis extension to post hospital discharge

Many stroke patients do not recover full mobility at hospital discharge, and a significant number are discharged to a nursing home or a long-term acute care center (LTAC). Whether chemoprophylaxis should be continued after hospital discharge is unknown. A recently published retrospective cross-sectional analysis showed that up to 1.9% of stroke patients in the USA are discharged on some form of VTE prophylaxis, with Apixaban and Rivaroxaban being the most commonly used agents [22]. This very small percentage is not surprising, as currently available guidelines recommend stopping chemoprophylaxis for stroke patients at hospital discharge, regardless of their mobility state or disposition. However, a recently published systematic review and meta-analysis showed a VTE incidence reduction benefit in acute ischemic stroke patients who received extended chemoprophylaxis (for 4 to 5 weeks) with a minor increase in the risk of major bleeding [23]. Although composite outcomes from different studies were included in this analysis, and despite some patients receiving extended chemoprophylaxis while still hospitalized, this study highlights the need for randomized trials, probably targeting stroke patients without full recovery at discharge.

2.2.4 VTE diagnosis in stroke patients

The diagnosis of VTE in critical care patients is usually challenging. Intubated, sedated patients cannot report limb or chest pain, and stroke patients with aphasia face the same issue. Additionally, medical equipment covering their bodies, such as warmers, coolers, or ICP monitors, can sometimes hinder a proper physical exam. Physicians should be vigilant and actively look for VTE at every patient encounter.

Several studies have investigated the benefit of regular interval screening for VTE in these patients, regardless of the presence of any signs or symptoms. One study screened asymptomatic, non-ambulatory neurosurgical hospitalized patients using venous duplex ultrasound. Despite all patients being on mechanical prophylaxis and the majority receiving chemoprophylaxis, the DVT incidence was about 23% [24]. Two other studies found that elevated D-dimer was an independent significant factor for the presence of VTE in stroke patients at admission [25] and during hospitalization [26], suggesting the use of D-dimer for initial screening and selection of patients in whom further diagnostic imaging might be helpful.

Although current guidelines do not recommend regular screening for VTE in asymptomatic patients, venous ultrasound is non-invasive, safe, and relatively inexpensive, and could potentially prevent VTE complications.

2.2.5 Chemical vs. mechanical prophylaxis

Although chemical VTE prophylaxis is superior to mechanical prophylaxis [27], mechanical prophylaxis is an attractive alternative in patients with a contraindication to chemical prophylaxis. Several types of devices are available with the most commonly used being intermittent pneumatic compression (IPC) and graduated compressive stockings (GCS). The use of such devices is not without its caveats. IPCs mimic the skeletal muscles by creating a pulsatile blood flow in the legs' deep veins, while GCS increase their venous flow and velocity [28]. It is almost universally agreed that IPCs are superior to GCS, and the latter should not be used in stroke patients [15]. Both the Canadian stroke guidelines and the American Society of Hematology guidelines for VTE management do not recommend combing chemical and mechanical prophylaxis over chemical prophylaxis alone [15, 27]. However, a meta-analysis published in 2016 found a moderate level of evidence supporting the combination of chemical and mechanical prophylaxis over IPC alone or anticoagulation alone for VTE prevention [29]. Contraindications for IPC use include the presence of limb ischemia due to peripheral vascular disease, severe limb edema, lung ulcers, or the presence of a DVT.

2.2.6 VTE treatment in stroke patients

VTE treatment, on the other hand, is not specific to stroke patients and follows the treatment algorithms used for other patients. Initiation of treatment is usually a clinical decision and depends on the risk of hemorrhagic transformation. This decision-making process involves assessing the patient's overall clinical status, including factors such as the size and location of the thrombus, the patient's hemodynamic stability, and the potential for bleeding complications.

Although the majority of VTEs develop during hospitalization, some patients presenting with acute ischemic stroke are found to have VTE upon admission [30]. As screening for DVT is part of every stroke workup, stroke patients with confirmed DVT on admission may be diagnosed with cryptogenic stroke due to paradoxical emboli. Subsequently, an extensive workup will be performed to locate a patent foramen ovale, an atrial septal defect, or pulmonary arteriovenous malformations through which the thrombus might have migrated from the venous to the arterial circulation [15]. Therefore, the presence of VTE at the time of stroke admission can complicate clinical management and necessitate a tailored approach to treatment.

In hemodynamically stable patients, stroke treatment is initially prioritized over VTE treatment. This is because the immediate goal is to restore cerebral perfusion and minimize neurological damage. Starting patients on therapeutic anticoagulation in addition to dual antiplatelet therapy presents a significantly high risk of bleeding, whether intra- or extracranial. This requires a multidisciplinary approach and careful monitoring to ensure the best possible care for stroke patients with concurrent VTE.

In hemodynamically unstable patients due to massive acute PE, tissue plasminogen activator (tPA) is indicated. If patients are deemed high risk for tPA due to the risk of hemorrhagic conversion or extracranial bleed, a catheter or surgical embolectomy should be performed [31].

Patients with VTE who receive tPA for their stroke warrant repeated imaging to confirm the resolution or persistence of the VTE and guide further treatment decisions. If the VTE persists, alternative anticoagulation strategies may be considered, balancing the risk of recurrent thromboembolism with the potential for hemorrhagic complications.

Such strategies might include delaying the initiation of therapeutic anticoagulation, particularly in patients with large ischemic strokes, usually for a period of 1 to 2 weeks. Meanwhile, an inferior vena cava (IVC) filter should be immediately placed until therapeutic anticoagulation can be started. Other strategies include using a single antiplatelet agent instead of dual therapy along with therapeutic anticoagulation, especially in patients with mild to moderate ischemic infarcts and limited intracranial atherosclerosis, or using anticoagulation alone without antiplatelet agents, particularly when the origin of the stroke is embolic [15].

Many physicians choose continuous intravenous infusion of UFH as the anticoagulant of choice for VTE treatment in this subset of patients, mainly due to the availability of an effective reversal agent (protamine sulfate) and the relative ease of stopping the infusion if a hemorrhagic complication occurs. After the initiation of anticoagulation, it might be prudent to repeat brain imaging, usually with a head CT, typically done 24 hours after therapeutic anticoagulation has been achieved. It is also recommended to keep these patients closely monitored with frequent neurological exams until the risk period has lapsed. Treatment duration will depend on the perceived cause of the VTE [32].

Many patients will be switched to direct oral anticoagulants (DOACs) upon discharge. Careful consideration is required when treating patients with antiphospholipid syndrome, as vitamin K antagonists are recommended over DOACs for the treatment of VTE [32].

When compared to other patient populations, stroke patients with upper extremity hemiplegia are theoretically at increased risk of upper extremity DVT. Treatment duration is usually 3 months. However, if the DVT is associated with a central venous catheter that has not been removed, treatment is continued until the catheter is removed, with a minimum duration of 3 months [32].

2.3 VTE in patients with acute intracranial bleed

Compared to patients with TBI or acute ischemic stroke, there is significantly less data and research available on the prophylaxis and treatment of VTE in patients with acute intracranial bleed. The remainder of this chapter will discuss the available data on patients with aneurysmal subarachnoid hemorrhage (aSAH) and spontaneous intraparenchymal bleed.

2.3.1 Aneurysmal subarachnoid hemorrhage

Subarachnoid hemorrhage due to a ruptured aneurysm is an increasing cause of intracranial bleeding. Affected patients typically require a prolonged hospital stay, regardless of the condition's severity. They are usually monitored for cerebral vasospasm in a critical care setting with frequent neurological checks. This extended hospital stay, usually lasting for a couple of weeks, coupled with various neurological deficits, puts them at a significantly higher risk for VTE development.

Many physicians are uncomfortable starting VTE chemoprophylaxis for these patients, fearing it may worsen their intracranial bleed. However, almost all published research and guidelines suggest starting chemical prophylaxis 24 hours after the aneurysm has been secured (either by coiling or surgically) [33]. This aligns with other published research showing no increased risk of craniotomy after initiating VTE prophylaxis before 48 hours [34]. Notably, patients requiring an EVD (External Ventricular Drainage) or mechanical ventilation had a higher rate of symptomatic VTEs [35], and VTEs peeked between day 5 and day 9 after hospital admission [36].

The scarcity of published data on the initiation of therapeutic anticoagulation in patients with aSAH necessitates a case-by-case approach to treating VTE, potentially including the use of an IVC filter until a decision to initiate therapeutic anticoagulation is made. However, having a secured aneurysm and serial head CT scans facilitates the decision to initiate and continue therapeutic anticoagulation [37].

2.3.2 Spontaneous intraparenchymal bleed

Although very few randomized controlled trials have been published about the use of VTE prophylactic anticoagulation in patients with spontaneous intraparenchymal bleed, all published data and guidelines agree that chemoprophylaxis is safe and effective, as it reduces VTE incidence and mortality without incurring additional bleeding risk [38–40]. IPCs should be started on the day of admission, and LMWH or UFH is ideally started within 48 hours, after confirming a stable hematoma, usually with a plain head CT [33, 41]. Later initiation of LMWH (at the 72-hour mark) did not show a reduced risk of hematoma expansion, thus proving that earlier initiation of LMWH is safe [42].

Since the management of patients with spontaneous intraparenchymal bleed typically does not involve surgical intervention, physicians are often hesitant to initiate VTE prophylaxis. This phenomenon was demonstrated in a study published in 2015, which showed that only 16.5% of patients with spontaneous intracranial hemorrhage received VTE chemoprophylaxis during their hospital stay, with half of these patients starting anticoagulation on day 2 [43]. This highlights the need for clearer guidelines and more proactive approaches to VTE prevention in this patient population.

Treating thromboembolism in such patients consistently sparks debates among treating physicians. The absence of randomized controlled trials and the significant variability in VTE treatment initiation dates in patients with intraparenchymal bleed, which range from 2.5 days to 18 weeks as reported in the literature [44], further complicates the issue. Consequently, physicians must rely on their clinical judgment and experience, often considering patient-specific factors and the potential risks and benefits of early versus delayed treatment. The location of bleeding may influence the decision on when to initiate therapeutic anticoagulation. It has been demonstrated that lobar bleeds carry a higher risk of hematoma expansion following the initiation of therapeutic anticoagulation with DOACs, compared to deep bleeds [45]. The presence of a stable hematoma might also influence the decision [46]. An IVC filter might be a temporary solution until therapeutic anticoagulation is started.

3. Conclusion

In the end, starting anticoagulation for critically ill patients requires a holistic approach, considering comorbidities not discussed above, such as extracranial bleeding, thrombocytopenia, coagulation disorders, and more. Ultimately, this decision is made on a case-by-case basis, typically involving a collaborative decision between the intensivist and the neurologist. In tertiary care centers, this often includes input from neurointensivists and stroke specialists.

Acknowledgements

Artificial intelligence (AI) through Microsoft Copilot was utilized to correct English and grammar mistakes.

Conflict of interest

The author declares no conflict of interest.

Author details

Mostafa A. AL Turk
Pulmonary and NeuroCritical Care, Bellevue Medical Center, Beirut, Lebanon

*Address all correspondence to: mostafaturk@hotmail.com

References

[1] Yeates EO, Grigorian A, Schubl SD, Kuza CM, Joe V, Lekawa M, et al. Chemoprophylaxis and venous thromboembolism in traumatic brain injury at different trauma centers. The American Surgeon. 2020;**86**(4):362-368

[2] Grosse SD, Nelson RE, Nyarko KA, Richardson LC, Raskob GE. The economic burden of incident venous thromboembolism in the United States: A review of estimated attributable healthcare costs. Thrombosis Research. 2016;**137**:3-10

[3] Skrifvars MB, Bailey M, Presneill J, French C, Nichol A, Little L, et al. Venous thromboembolic events in critically ill traumatic brain injury patients. Intensive Care Medicine. 2017;**43**(3):419-428

[4] Zhang M, Parikh B, Dirlikov B, Cage T, Lee M, Singh H. Elevated risk of venous thromboembolism among post-traumatic brain injury patients requiring pharmaceutical immobilization. Journal of Clinical Neuroscience. 2020;**75**:66-70

[5] Cole KL, Nguyen S, Gelhard S, Hardy J, Cortez J, Nunez JM, et al. Factors associated with venous thromboembolism development in patients with traumatic brain injury. Neurocritical Care. 2024;**40**(2):568-576

[6] Mohseni S, Talving P, Lam L, Chan LS, Ives C, Demetriades D. Venous thromboembolic events in isolated severe traumatic brain injury. Journal of Emergencies, Trauma, and Shock. 2012;**5**(1):11-15

[7] Byrne JP, Mason SA, Gomez D, Hoeft C, Subacius H, Xiong W, et al. Timing of pharmacologic venous thromboembolism prophylaxis in severe traumatic brain injury: A propensity-matched cohort study. Journal of the American College of Surgeons. 2016;**223**(4):621-31 e5

[8] Hollfelder EK, Rappaport S, Cheng J, Patel JH. Retrospective evaluation of chemical venous thromboembolism prophylaxis in traumatic brain injury. Surgery in Practice and Science. 2023;**13**:100168

[9] Carney N, Totten AM, O'Reilly C, Ullman JS, Hawryluk GW, Bell MJ, et al. Guidelines for the management of severe traumatic brain injury, Fourth Edition. Neurosurgery. 2017;**80**(1):6-15

[10] Minshall CT, Eriksson EA, Leon SM, Doben AR, McKinzie BP, Fakhry SM. Safety and efficacy of heparin or enoxaparin prophylaxis in blunt trauma patients with a head abbreviated injury severity score >2. The Journal of Trauma. 2011;**71**(2):396-399; discussion 9-400

[11] van Erp IA, Gaitanidis A, El Moheb M, Kaafarani HMA, Saillant N, Duhaime AC, et al. Low-molecular-weight heparin versus unfractionated heparin in pediatric traumatic brain injury. Journal of Neurosurgery. Pediatrics. 2021;**27**(4):469-474

[12] Cho YW, Scrushy M, Zhu M, DeAtkine E, Zhu M, Wan B, et al. Early administration of high dose enoxaparin after traumatic brain injury. European Journal of Trauma and Emergency Surgery. 2023;**49**(5):2295-2303

[13] Khan MT, Ikram A, Saeed O, Afridi T, Sila CA, Smith MS, et al. Deep vein thrombosis in acute stroke - a systemic review of the literature. Cureus. 2017;**9**(12):e1982

[14] Gao X, Zeng L, Wang H, Zeng S, Tian J, Chen L, et al. Prevalence of

venous thromboembolism in intensive care units: A meta-analysis. Journal of Clinical Medicine. 2022;**11**(22):6691

[15] Heran M, Lindsay P, Gubitz G, Yu A, Ganesh A, Lund R, et al. Canadian stroke best practice recommendations: Acute stroke management, 7(th) edition practice guidelines update, 2022. The Canadian Journal of Neurological Sciences. 2024;**51**(1):1-31

[16] Powers WJ, Rabinstein AA, Ackerson T, Adeoye OM, Bambakidis NC, Becker K, et al. Guidelines for the early management of patients with acute ischemic stroke: 2019 update to the 2018 guidelines for the early management of acute ischemic stroke: A guideline for healthcare professionals from the American heart association/American stroke association. Stroke. 2019;**50**(12):e344-e418

[17] Al Turk M, Abraham M. Incidence of symptomatic venous thromboembolisms in stroke patients. Journal of Intensive Care Medicine. 2024;**39**(9):895-899

[18] Crowther MA, Petr K, Peng L, Frank C, Leslie BB, Anthony CKC. Significant differences in neutralization of heparin and its low molecular fragments by protamine sulfate: An *in vivo* study. Blood. 2004;**104**(11):1850

[19] Bozic-Mijovski M, Vucnik M, Boc V, Blinc A, Stegnar M. Ex vivo neutralization of unfractionated heparin for assessing overall haemostatic potential in patient plasma. Thrombosis Research. 2015;**135**(5):1042-1044

[20] Baruch D, Lindhout T, Wagenvoord R, Hemker HC. Inhibition of thrombin-catalyzed reactions in blood coagulation and platelet activation by heparin fractions in the absence of antithrombin III. Haemostasis. 1986;**16**(2):71-81

[21] Samama MM, Bara L, Gerotziafas GT. Mechanisms for the antithrombotic activity in man of low molecular weight heparins (LMWHs). Haemostasis. 1994;**24**(2):105-117

[22] Dawwas GK, Cuker A, Rothstein A, Hennessy S. Trends in post-discharge prophylactic anticoagulant use among stroke patients in the United States between 2006 and 2019. Journal of Stroke and Cerebrovascular Diseases. 2022;**31**(10):106700

[23] Valeriani E, Potere N, Candeloro M, Spoto S, Porreca E, Rutjes AW, et al. Extended venous thromboprophylaxis in patients hospitalized for acute ischemic stroke: A systematic review and meta-analysis. European Journal of Internal Medicine. 2022;**95**:80-86

[24] Dermody M, Alessi-Chinetti J, Iafrati MD, Estes JM. The utility of screening for deep venous thrombosis in asymptomatic, non-ambulatory neurosurgical patients. Journal of Vascular Surgery. 2011;**53**(5):1309-1315

[25] Mori T, Yoshioka K, Tanno Y. Frequency of deep vein thrombosis at admission for acute stroke and associated factors: A cross-sectional study. Thrombosis Journal. 2021;**19**(1):62

[26] Kelly J, Rudd A, Lewis RR, Coshall C, Parmar K, Moody A, et al. Screening for proximal deep vein thrombosis after acute ischemic stroke: A prospective study using clinical factors and plasma D-dimers. Journal of Thrombosis and Haemostasis. 2004;**2**(8):1321-1326

[27] Schunemann HJ, Cushman M, Burnett AE, Kahn SR, Beyer-Westendorf J, Spencer FA, et al. American Society of Hematology 2018 guidelines for management of venous thromboembolism: Prophylaxis for hospitalized and nonhospitalized

medical patients. Blood Advances. 2018;**2**(22):3198-3225

[28] Herring B, Lowen D, Ho P, Hodgson R. A systematic review of venous thromboembolism mechanical prophylaxis devices during surgery. Langenbeck's Archives of Surgery. 2023;**408**(1):410

[29] Kakkos SK, Caprini JA, Geroulakos G, Nicolaides AN, Stansby G, Reddy DJ, et al. Combined intermittent pneumatic leg compression and pharmacological prophylaxis for prevention of venous thromboembolism. Cochrane Database of Systematic Reviews. 2016;**9**(9):CD005258

[30] Windecker S, Stortecky S, Meier B. Paradoxical embolism. Journal of the American College of Cardiology. 2014;**64**(4):403-415

[31] Konstantinides SV, Meyer G, Becattini C, Bueno H, Geersing GJ, Harjola VP, et al. 2019 ESC guidelines for the diagnosis and management of acute pulmonary embolism developed in collaboration with the European Respiratory Society (ERS). European Heart Journal. 2020;**41**(4):543-603

[32] Stevens SM, Woller SC, Baumann Kreuziger L, Doerschug K, Geersing GJ, Klok FA, et al. Antithrombotic therapy for VTE disease: Compendium and review of CHEST guidelines 2012-2021. Chest. 2024;**166**(2):388-404

[33] Nyquist P, Bautista C, Jichici D, Burns J, Chhangani S, DeFilippis M, et al. Prophylaxis of venous thrombosis in neurocritical care patients: An evidence-based guideline: A statement for healthcare professionals from the neurocritical care society. Neurocritical Care. 2016;**24**(1):47-60

[34] Jakob DA, Lewis M, Benjamin ER, Mitchao DP, Exadaktylos AK, Demetriades D. Timing of venous thromboembolic pharmacological prophylaxis in traumatic combined subdural and subarachnoid hemorrhage. American Journal of Surgery. 2022;**223**(6):1194-1199

[35] Kilgore CB, Nair SK, Ran KR, Caplan JM, Jackson CM, Gonzalez LF, et al. Venous thromboembolism in aneurysmal subarachnoid hemorrhage: Risk factors and timing of chemoprophylaxis. Clinical Neurology and Neurosurgery. 2023;**231**:107822

[36] Liang CW, Su K, Liu JJ, Dogan A, Hinson HE. Timing of deep vein thrombosis formation after aneurysmal subarachnoid hemorrhage. Journal of Neurosurgery. 2015;**123**(4):891-896

[37] Pandit S, Dube SK, Sokhal S, Chaturvedi A. Management of ruptured intracranial aneurysm with DVT: Case report and brief review of literature. Journal of Neuroanaesthesiology and Critical Care. 2024 (EFirst)

[38] Zhou Y, Wang G, Xue C, He G, Zhang Y, He F, et al. Effect of heparin for the prevention of venous thromboembolism in patients with spontaneous intracranial cerebral hemorrhage: A meta analysis. Therapeutic Advances in Drug Safety. 2024;**15**:1-13

[39] Sprugel MI, Sembill JA, Kuramatsu JB, Gerner ST, Hagen M, Roeder SS, et al. Heparin for prophylaxis of venous thromboembolism in intracerebral haemorrhage. Journal of Neurology, Neurosurgery, and Psychiatry. 2019;**90**(7):783-791

[40] Paciaroni M, Agnelli G, Alberti A, Becattini C, Guercini F, Martini G, et al. PREvention of VENous thromboembolism in hemorrhagic stroke patients - preventihs study:

A randomized controlled trial and a systematic review and meta-analysis. European Neurology. 2020;**83**(6):566-575

[41] Dong C, Li Y, Ma MZ. Venous thromboembolism prophylaxis after spontaneous intracerebral hemorrhage: A review. The Neurologist. 2024;**29**(1):54-58

[42] Qian C, Huhtakangas J, Juvela S, Bode MK, Tatlisumak T, Savolainen M, et al. Early vs. late enoxaparin for the prevention of venous thromboembolism in patients with ICH: A double blind placebo controlled multicenter study. Clinical Neurology and Neurosurgery. 2021;**202**:106534

[43] Prabhakaran S, Herbers P, Khoury J, Adeoye O, Khatri P, Ferioli S, et al. Is prophylactic anticoagulation for deep venous thrombosis common practice after intracerebral hemorrhage? Stroke. 2015;**46**(2):369-375

[44] Cai Q, Zhang X, Chen H. Patients with venous thromboembolism after spontaneous intracerebral hemorrhage: A review. Thrombosis Journal. 2021;**19**(1):93

[45] Eckman MH, Rosand J, Knudsen KA, Singer DE, Greenberg SM. Can patients be anticoagulated after intracerebral hemorrhage? A decision analysis. Stroke. 2003;**34**(7):1710-1716

[46] Hemphill JC 3rd, Greenberg SM, Anderson CS, Becker K, Bendok BR, Cushman M, et al. Guidelines for the Management of Spontaneous Intracerebral Hemorrhage: A guideline for healthcare professionals from the American heart association/ American stroke association. Stroke. 2015;**46**(7):2032-2060

Chapter 5

Management of Prostate Cancer Associated Disseminated Intravascular Coagulation (DIC): A Multidisciplinary and Individualized Approach

William Schwartzman, Parker Wilson, Zane Gray and Jue Wang

Abstract

Disseminated intravascular coagulation (DIC) is a complex clinical syndrome characterized by systemic activation of coagulation pathways, leading to the formation of microvascular thrombi, which can result in multi-organ dysfunction and bleeding due to the consumption of coagulation factors and platelets. In patients with prostate cancer, DIC poses a significant diagnostic and management challenge due to its multifactorial etiology, overlapping clinical features with other coagulopathies, and its impact on patient outcomes. DIC often presents with non-specific symptoms that overlap with those of advanced prostate cancer and its treatments, which may lead to delays in diagnosis. While the prognosis for prostate cancer patients with DIC is generally poor, active cancer therapy, including androgen deprivation therapy (ADT), chemotherapy, and newer anticancer therapies can improve overall survival by addressing the underlying malignancy. Understanding the interplay between prostate cancer progression and hypercoagulation provides a foundation for developing individualized precision medicine strategies to prevent and manage DIC in prostate cancer patients, potentially improving outcomes in this challenging clinical scenario. Future research will continue to refine these approaches, integrating new discoveries into personalized care strategies that address both the malignancy and its hematologic complications.

Keywords: prostate cancer, disseminated intravascular coagulation (DIC), diagnosis, prognosis, management, genetic alterations, individualized approach, precision medicine, outcome

1. Introduction

Prostate cancer is the most diagnosed cancer in men and is the second leading cause of cancer-related deaths in men each year [1]. At diagnosis, most patients have

IntechOpen

localized disease. However, 5–6% of patients are diagnosed with metastatic disease and 30–40% of patients will develop biochemical recurrence after definitive treatment (surgery and/or radiotherapy). A substantial proportion of these patients will develop metastatic prostate cancer. The mainstream treatment of prostate cancer remains androgen deprivation therapy (ADT) given the nature of the disease. However, with progression of disease, the hormone sensitive prostate cancer could develop into castration resistant prostate cancer despite ADT in the long term with more cancer related complications [2]. Prostate cancer can lead to the activation of coagulation cascade which could present as a spectrum ranging from clinically asymptomatic, only with laboratory markers of coagulation activation, to the extreme case of disseminated intravascular coagulation (DIC) manifesting as treatment-resistant thrombosis or life-threatening bleeding. The pathophysiology of DIC involves widespread activation of the coagulation cascade, leading to the formation of microthrombi throughout the vasculature, which can result in organ dysfunction and bleeding due to the consumption of clotting factors and platelets [3]. While DIC is a rare manifestation in prostate cancer, its occurrence signifies a poor prognosis and presents significant diagnostic and management challenges due to the complex interplay between cancer progression, coagulopathy, and treatment-related factors [3–6]. Better understanding of the epidemiology, pathophysiology, diagnosis, and management of DIC in the context of prostate cancer is crucial for improving patient care.

2. Epidemiology

The incidence of DIC in prostate cancer is not well-defined due to its rarity and often subclinical presentation. However, DIC in metastatic prostate cancer is likely underrecognized and underdiagnosed due to several factors (**Table 1**). The clinical

Diagnostic challenges	**Common causes**
Non-Specific Symptoms	Early symptoms of DIC, such as mild bleeding (e.g., epistaxis) or thrombosis, can be non-specific and easily attributed to other conditions, leading to delayed recognition
Overlap with Cancer Symptoms	Symptoms of DIC can overlap with those of advanced prostate cancer, such as fatigue, weight loss, and general malaise, making it challenging to distinguish between the two conditions.
Laboratory Test Limitations	Routine coagulation tests may not always clearly indicate DIC, especially in the early stages.
Complex Pathophysiology	The pathophysiology of DIC in prostate cancer involves complex interactions between tumor-derived factors and the coagulation system, which can complicate the diagnosis.
Lack of Awareness	There may be a lack of awareness or suspicion among clinicians regarding the association between DIC and prostate cancer, particularly in cases where DIC is the initial manifestation of prostate cancer.
Diagnostic Challenges	In patients with advanced or metastatic prostate cancer, the presence of multiple comorbidities and the effects of prior treatments can obscure the clinical picture, making the diagnosis of DIC more challenging.

Table 1.
Common causes for delay in diagnosis or misdiagnosis of disseminated intravascular coagulation (DIC) in prostate cancer.

presentation of DIC in prostate cancer patients is often less acute and more insidious compared to DIC associated with conditions like sepsis or trauma. This can lead to a more chronic and subclinical progression, where the initial symptoms may be subtle or nonspecific, such as mild thrombocytopenia or elevated D-dimer levels, which can also result from prostate cancer involvement of the bone marrow and treatment related adverse events. Moreover, the pathophysiology of DIC in prostate cancer involves complex interactions between tumor cells and the coagulation system, including the role of extracellular vesicles exposing tissue factor, which may not be routinely assessed in clinical practice. Over the past two decades, the number of case reports documenting DIC in prostate cancer has indeed increased. This rise is likely due to a combination of increased awareness of this rare but serious complication and the development of more effective cancer therapies that allow patients to live longer. As patients survive longer due to advancements in treatment options, there are more opportunities to observe complications like DIC that might have previously gone unnoticed. This also highlights the importance of careful monitoring and timely intervention in managing coagulopathy in prostate cancer patients [6].

A retrospective analysis by Hyman et al. identified 42 prostate cancer patients with DIC and excessive fibrinolysis (DIC XFL) [4]. The common risk factors for DIC in prostate cancer patients include high Gleason Score, advanced disease stage, castration-resistant prostate cancer, prior chemotherapy, and surgical intervention. Most of these patients had high-grade prostate cancer, with 26% having a Gleason score of 7 and 45% having a Gleason score of 8–10. Most cases of DIC occurred in the setting of metastatic disease, with 93% of patients being resistant to castration and 50% having received prior chemotherapy. In a study of 85 patients by Ni and Wang, the median age was 68 years (range, 44–92 years) [6]. Most patients (98%) have adenocarcinoma, two (2%) patients with small cell carcinoma. The median of PSA was 614 ng/ml (range: 0.8–8138). A Gleason score of 8 or higher was found in 67% of patients. Distant metastasis was reported in 98% of patients.

3. Pathophysiology of DIC in prostate cancer

The development of DIC in prostate cancer is a multifactorial process (**Table 2**). Tissue factor (TF) plays a critical role in the coagulation system and is significantly implicated in the pathophysiology of DIC in the setting of prostate cancer. TF is a transmembrane glycoprotein that initiates the extrinsic pathway of coagulation by binding to Factor VII/VIIa, leading to thrombin generation and fibrin clot formation [6]. The overexpression of TF in prostate cancer, particularly in the advanced stages of disease leads to increased procoagulant activity and contributes to the hypercoagulable state observed in these patients. Elevated levels of extracellular vesicle-associated TF have been documented in prostate cancer patients with DIC, indicating that tumor-derived EVs exposing TF play a significant role in the development of DIC [7–11]. The interaction between tumor-derived EVs, monocytes, and platelets further amplifies TF activity, promoting coagulation and contributing to the systemic activation of the coagulation cascade seen in DIC. This mechanism underscores the intrinsic relationship between cancer progression and coagulation abnormalities, as controlling the underlying malignancy often leads to an improvement in DIC.

Prostate cancer, particularly in its metastatic form, is associated with increased expression of factors like cancer procoagulant (CP), which has direct thrombin-like activity, further contributing to the hypercoagulable state [12]. Moreover, metastatic

	Molecular mechanism
Tumor-Derived Factors	Extracellular vesicles (EVs) from prostate cancer cells with high TF expression exhibit significant pro-coagulant activity, promoting thrombin generation and correlating with the oncogenic and metastatic potential of the cells.
Inflammatory Cytokines	Pro-inflammatory cytokines (IL-6, TNF-α, IL-1β) activate endothelial cells and monocytes, increasing procoagulant factors.
Genetic and Epigenetic Alterations	TF expression is regulated by oncogenes and environmental factors, and tumor-derived TF-positive EVs are associated with increased thrombin generation and cancer progression. DNA methylation and histone modifications alter the expression of procoagulant and anticoagulant genes.
Tumor Microenvironment	Cancer-stromal cell interactions lead to the secretion of pro-inflammatory and procoagulant factors.
Platelet Activation	Altered megakaryocyte function in bone marrow leads to platelets with increased procoagulant properties. Direct interactions activate platelets, releasing procoagulant factors and microparticles.

Table 2.
The molecular mechanisms and insights into DIC in prostate cancer.

involvement of the bone marrow can lead to the release of procoagulant substances, while liver metastases or other organ dysfunctions can impair the clearance of activated clotting factors, exacerbating the coagulopathic process. Addition, inflammatory cytokines released by the tumor or in response to treatment can enhance coagulation. Tumor invasion and metastasis can lead to endothelial damage, further promoting coagulation. The resulting imbalance between coagulation and fibrinolysis leads to the characteristic features of DIC: thrombosis in small and medium-sized vessels and consumption of platelets and coagulation factors, which predispose patients to bleeding [13].

Prostate cancer patients, even in early stages, may exhibit a hypercoagulable state. Invasive procedures such as prostate biopsy can exacerbate coagulation disorders in early-stage prostate cancer [11]. In advanced prostate cancer, this hypercoagulable state can progress to DIC. The increased tumor burden seen in metastatic castrate resistant prostate cancer (mCRPC) correlates with higher levels of these procoagulant factors, leading to more severe DIC. This is because larger or more aggressive tumors release more EVs, which in turn increases systemic procoagulant activity. This heightened procoagulant state results in the formation of microthrombi, consumption of clotting factors, and subsequent bleeding complications, all of which are hallmarks of severe DIC [7, 9, 10].

DIC is a complex coagulopathy characterized by systemic activation of coagulation pathways, leading to the consumption of coagulation factors and platelets, and a concurrent process of hyperfibrinolysis. The degree of fibrinolytic activation in DIC varies, resulting in three distinct types: DIC with suppressed fibrinolysis, DIC with enhanced fibrinolysis, and an intermediate type known as balanced fibrinolysis. DIC with enhanced fibrinolysis is the least common subtype and is notably linked to prostate cancer. This subtype is characterized by massive thrombin generation combined with systemic pathologic hyperfibrinolysis, leading to severe bleeding due to excessive plasmin formation [4, 14–16].

4. Diagnosis

The clinical diagnosis of DIC involves recognizing a constellation of signs and symptoms, supported by laboratory findings [15–19]. These include prolonged prothrombin time (PT), activated partial thromboplastin time (aPTT), low fibrinogen levels, and elevated D-dimer levels. However, these laboratory abnormalities are non-specific and therefore must be interpreted in the context of the patient's overall clinical picture. DIC in prostate cancer may present with symptoms such as bleeding (mucosal bleeding, hematuria, gastrointestinal bleeding, or intracranial hemorrhage), thrombosis (e.g., deep vein thrombosis, pulmonary embolism, or arterial thrombosis), and purpura, petechiae, and signs of organ dysfunction (including renal failure, hepatic dysfunction, and respiratory distress) [4–6] all of which are non-specific findings and can be attributed to other etiologies, particularly in cancer patients who may already have a tendency for bleeding or clotting abnormalities. The constitutive symptoms of DIC, such as fatigue, shortness of breath, and bleeding, can overlap with the symptoms of advanced prostate cancer or its treatments. This complexity contributes to diagnostic challenges and delays in diagnosis if clinicians do not maintain a high index of suspicion (**Table 3**). For instance, thrombocytopenia in a prostate cancer patient might be attributed to chemotherapy or bone marrow infiltration by metastatic cancer, rather than DIC.

Ni and Wang characterized the presentation of 85 patients presenting with DIC and prostate cancer [6]. At diagnosis of DIC, the median platelet count was 75 $*10^9$ /L (range: 3–205). Regarding the presenting symptoms of DIC, subcutaneous bleeding was reported in 64% of cases; hematuria in 27%. Invasive procedures including prostate biopsy might have been the provoking events of DIC in 25% of the cases. Bleeding induced by DIC included subcutaneous bleeding in 52 patients (64%), hematuria in 22 (27%), epistaxis in 21 (26%), invasive procedure (incision, biopsy, trauma, operation) bleeding in 20 (25%), gastrointestinal bleeding in 18 (22%), oral in 13 (16%), and cerebral bleeding in 6 (7%).

Differential diagnosis	Key clinical and laboratory features	Distinguishing factors from DIC
Primary Fibrinolysis	Bleeding tendencies, elevated D dimer, low fibrinogen	Lacks widespread microvascular thrombosis seen in DIC
Thrombocytopenias of Diverse Etiologies	Low platelet counts, bleeding	Normal D-dimer, usually normal PT/aPTT
Thrombotic Microangiopathies (TMAs)	Thrombocytopenia, microangiopathic hemolytic anemia, organ dysfunction	Typically no significant coagulation factor consumption as seen in DIC
Sepsis	Systemic inflammatory response syndrome (SIRS) criteria, potential coagulopathy	Need to distinguish if coagulopathy is due to infection or underlying malignancy
Liver Disease	Prolonged PT/aPTT, low fibrinogen, signs of hepatic dysfunction	No microvascular thrombosis, additional signs of liver dysfunction
Vasculitis	Bleeding and thrombosis, signs of systemic inflammation	Specific laboratory markers and signs of systemic inflammation

Table 3.
The differential diagnoses of DIC in patients with prostate cancer.

5. Management of DIC in prostate cancer

Management of DIC in prostate cancer remains challenging due to the inherent biologic heterogeneity of prostate cancer, its varied clinical presentations, and the lack of evidence-based treatment strategies. The central dogma behind the treatment of DIC is to treat the underlying etiology, which is made more difficult in relapsed prostate cancer by the limited options and potential side effects of cancer therapies, which can exacerbate thrombocytopenia or worsen coagulation abnormalities.

5.1 Anticancer therapy

No Randomized Control Trials (RCTs) have ever been done for the treatment of DIC in prostate cancer; however, case reports suggest the role of hormonal therapies, such as luteinizing hormone-releasing hormone (LHRH) agonists and antiandrogens, chemotherapy and radio-labeled treatments that can help reduce the overall disease burden and provide control or resolution of DIC in these patients [18–22].

In our previous study of 85 patients, individuals receiving cancer-directed therapy at the time of DIC had a significantly prolonged median overall survival (OS) of 12 months compared to 2 weeks in those receiving only best supportive care (BSC) ($p < 0.001$) [6]. In another study, the reversal of DIC with excessive fibrinolysis in prostate cancer patients was observed in 20% of metastatic patients who received new chemotherapy regimens. This intervention extended the median survival from 4 weeks to 26 weeks, indicating a significant improvement in outcomes with effective chemotherapy [4]. Feinstein reported [3] that prompt diagnosis and treatment of the underlying malignancy can result in the resolution of DIC. The study emphasizes that if the tumor is responsive to chemotherapy, a reasonable median survival can be achieved. The primary mechanism of survival benefits is likely due to the effective control of the underlying malignancy, which also reduces the procoagulant activity of cancer cells and mitigates the hypercoagulable state associated with DIC.

The most critical issue in managing DIC in prostate cancer is the need for prompt diagnosis and the careful weighing of treatment options in a rapidly evolving and life-threatening situation. The decision-making process in such cases is indeed challenging due to the narrow window for intervention, where oncologists must balance the risks and benefits of initiating cancer therapy against supportive care. Individual patient and tumor characteristics, along with the extent of disease and prior treatment history, often play a decisive role in determining whether to pursue aggressive interventions or prioritize supportive care measures. If chemotherapy is initiated, close monitoring of the patient's response and any adverse effects would be crucial. Managing DIC in prostate cancer requires a multidisciplinary approach involving close collaboration among oncologists, hematologists, critical care specialists, and other healthcare providers. This collaboration is essential for optimizing both cancer treatment and the management of coagulopathy, including the use of supportive measures such as platelet transfusions, fresh frozen plasma, and anticoagulants as appropriate. The team should regularly reassess the benefits versus risks of continuing or modifying therapy as the patient's condition changes.

Recurrent DIC in prostate cancer patients is a significant clinical challenge, largely driven by underlying risk factors such as cancer characteristics, progression, and disease burden. The recurrent nature of DIC is often linked to these predisposing factors, which can include baseline hematological abnormalities and the presence of DIC at the time of initial cancer diagnosis. As the disease progresses, these factors can exacerbate the risk, leading to recurrent episodes of DIC. DIC may serve as a possible indicator of progression or loss of efficacy of the cancer therapy. Fortunately, there has been a rapid expansion in treatment options for the management of metastatic prostate cancer since the publication of our previous study. Androgen receptor signaling inhibitors (ARSIs) offer potent androgen receptor blockade and can be effective in managing advanced prostate cancer, potentially providing an alternative to chemotherapy in some cases. Radium-223 is alpha-emitting radiopharmaceutical which specifically targets bone metastases, delivering localized radiation and can help manage bone pain and progression in metastatic prostate cancer. PSMA-targeted radioligand Lutetium177 is a novel approach by delivering radioactive isotopes directly to prostate cancer cells, providing another therapeutic option for patients with advanced disease [23].

The advent of cancer-agnostic therapies, which target specific molecular alterations regardless of the cancer's tissue of origin, offers new possibilities in this context. For example, targeting actionable mutations or pathways involved in both tumor progression and coagulation could provide a dual benefit—controlling the tumor and mitigating the coagulopathy. This approach is particularly promising for patients with rapidly progressive tumors where traditional therapies might not be effective. The ability to improve outcomes in these patients, even in the presence of refractory metastatic disease, represents a significant advancement in cancer care. By focusing on individualized treatment strategies that consider the unique aspects of each patient's disease and coagulopathy, oncologists can make more informed decisions that potentially improve both survival and quality of life.

5.2 Supportive care

The primary goals of supportive care in DIC for prostate cancer patients are to stabilize coagulation, manage bleeding and thrombotic complications, treat the underlying malignancy, and provide individualized care based on continuous monitoring. Supportive care should be individualized based on the patient's symptoms, laboratory results, and the severity of the coagulopathy [5, 22]. Continuous monitoring of coagulation parameters and clinical status is essential.

Patients with DIC often experience significant bleeding (e.g., subcutaneous bleeding, hematuria) and thrombotic complications, which can severely impact their quality of life. Managing these symptoms may involves the administration of blood products such as fresh frozen plasma (FFP), cryoprecipitate, and platelet transfusions to replenish depleted coagulation factors and platelets, thereby managing bleeding and stabilizing coagulation parameters [6, 17, 18, 24]. Antifibrinolytic agents like epsilon-aminocaproic acid can be used to manage excessive fibrinolysis in the setting of persistent bleeding; however, these agents are highly pro-thrombotic and must be used cautiously in the setting of DIC where microthrombi are being formed. In addition, doses of unfractionated heparin or low molecular weight heparin (LMWH) may be employed to prevent thrombosis, provided there is no significant bleeding risk and therapeutic doses can be used in patients with active thrombus; however these must be used cautiously [17, 18, 24–26].

6. Prognosis

The prognosis of DIC in prostate cancer varies significantly with the stage of the cancer. DIC is rare in early-stage prostate cancer and has a more favorable prognosis with appropriate management of both the underlying malignancy and the coagulopathy. Prompt diagnosis and treatment are crucial to improving outcomes. Effective treatment of the underlying malignancy often leads to an improvement in DIC, as controlling the cancer reduces the procoagulant activity driving the coagulopathy.

Since DIC is often seen in the terminal stages of the disease, where therapeutic options are limited, and patients are often too frail to undergo aggressive interventions, the prognosis for advanced prostate cancer patients with DIC is generally poor. Recent studies showed that active cancer therapy may improve survival in a subgroup of patients, which highlights the importance of aggressive treatment of the underlying malignancy to improve survival outcomes [4–6].

While aggressive treatment options are available and may be appropriate for some prostate cancer patients with DIC, palliative care and hospice provide essential alternatives that focus on quality of life and patient-centered care. For patients who prioritize comfort and dignity over the continuation of aggressive interventions, these services offer compassionate and comprehensive support. The decision to transition to palliative care or hospice should be guided by the patient's goals, values, and the clinical realities of their condition, ensuring that care is aligned with what matters most to the patient and their family.

7. Genomic insights into the interplay between oncogene, alteration, prostate cancer progression, hypercoagulation, and DIC

The interplay between oncogene alterations, genomic evolution, prostate cancer progression, hypercoagulation, and DIC is a complex process. The genetic mechanisms responsible for neoplastic transformation, progression, metastasis (activation of oncogenes and inactivation of tumor suppressor genes) directly induce the expression of genes controlling hemostasis. Alterations of oncogenes and tumor suppressor genes can lead to the release of pro-coagulant factors, such as tissue factor-containing extracellular vesicles, which initiate and propagate the coagulation cascade. This shift towards a hypercoagulable state, driven by the tumor's aggressive behavior, ultimately results in DIC [27–34]. The coagulation system's activation can also influence cancer cell behavior, potentially leading to further genetic and epigenetic changes that drive tumor evolution [28–33]. Activation of blood coagulation cascade results in a selective advantage for cancer cells, as fibrin provides a scaffold for anchorage and invasion, and coagulation proteins induce receptor-mediated intracellular signals promoting invasive growth. The procoagulant activity of cancer cells also share the core mechanisms of cancer onset and progression [30, 31].

8. Precision medicine approach

Given the limited treatment options often associated with late-stage disease, the need for biomarker-guided therapy selection is more critical than ever. The integration of genomic and clinical biomarkers into the management of DIC in prostate cancer allows for a more personalized and precise approach to therapy (**Table 4**). Recent studies demonstrate that the so-called 'castration-resistant' tumors are still dependent on androgen receptor signaling. Various molecular mechanisms (e.g., androgen receptor gene amplification, overexpression, AR Splice Variants (e.g., AR-V7) or mutations, enhanced AR signal transduction) have been reported in castration-resistant prostate

Biomarker	Drug class	Treatment options can be considered
Treatment naive	Androgen Deprivation Therapy (ADT)	Bicalutamide, Leuprolide, goserelin, and degarelix
Treatment naive	Androgen Receptor Pathway Inhibitors (ARPI)	Abiraterone acetate, enzalutamide, apalutamide, and darolutamide.
De Novo high risk metastatic prostate cancer	Combination Therapy	Triplet or Doublet Therapy
AR Amplification, AR-V7, PTEN, RB1 Aberrations	Chemotherapy	Docetaxel,cabazitaxel
Aggressive Variant Prostate Cancer	Chemotherapy	Docetaxel cabazitaxel Carboplatin plus cabazitaxel
Bone dominant metastasis	Radiopharmaceuticals	Radium-223 (Xofigo)
Prostate-specific membrane antigen (PSMA)	Radiopharmaceuticals	Pluvicto (lutetium Lu 177 vipivotide tetraxetan)
Homologous recombination repair gene mutations DNA Damage Repair (DDR) defects	PARP Inhibitors	Olaparib and rucaparib
Mismatch repair deficiency (dMMR) or microsatellite instability-high (MSI-H)	Anti-PD-1 antibody	Pembrolizumab
Mutational burden-high (TMB-H) [≥10 mutations/megabase (mut/Mb)]	Anti-PD-1 antibody	Pembrolizumab
NTRK gene fusions	Selective tropomyosin receptor kinase (TRK) inhibitor	Larotrectinib
HER2-positive (IHC3+)	Antibody-drug conjugate (ADC)	Trastuzumab deruxtecan

Table 4.
Biomarkers guide the selection of cancer therapy in patients with prostate cancer associated DIC.

cancers. AR amplification is a common mechanism of resistance in mCRPC, occurring in up to 80% of cases. Tumors with AR amplification are typically resistant to AR signaling inhibitors such as enzalutamide and apalutamide. Effective targeting of the androgen pathway in mCRPC often requires a combination of strategies, tailored to the specific molecular characteristics of the cancer [35]. Our observation of genetic alterations at the time of DIC in prostate cancer patients such as AR amplification provides insight on disease resistance and progression and help guide the selection of next-line therapies. For patients with AR amplification who progress on AR signaling inhibitors, switching to chemotherapy (e.g., docetaxel or cabazitaxel) may be beneficial. Additionally, ongoing research into novel agents targeting AR amplification and other resistance mechanisms continues to advance the therapeutic landscape for mCRPC. Similarly, the observation of gene amplifications of receptor tyrosine kinase at the onset of DIC in advanced prostate cancer mirrored previous findings [4, 32–34]. In patients with DIC, identifying these amplifications may prompt the use of targeted therapies that inhibit these pathways, potentially controlling tumor-driven coagulopathy [35]. Alterations in tumor suppressor genes such as TP53, PTEN and

RB1 are associated with more aggressive disease and poor prognosis. In the setting of DIC, these alterations may guide the use of chemotherapy or experimental therapies. The presence of multiple tumor suppressor gene alterations may indicate the need for combination therapy or enrollment in clinical trials exploring novel agents [36]. Defects in DNA damage repair (DDR) genes (e.g., BRCA1, BRCA2, ATM) are linked to a subset of prostate cancers with increased sensitivity to PARP inhibitors [37]. High TMB and MSI instability are markers of genomic instability and are associated with responsiveness to immunotherapy [38]. In prostate cancer patients with DIC, these markers may guide the use of immune checkpoint inhibitors, offering an alternative approach when conventional therapies are limited by coagulopathy.

The treatment paradigm for de novo high volume metastatic hormone-sensitive prostate cancer has evolved rapidly in the past decade with the approval of several life-prolonging therapies including docetaxel chemotherapy and multiple androgen receptor pathway inhibitors (ARPI). Treatment-naive patients with high-risk features should be considered for aggressive upfront therapy, including doublet or triplet therapy to maximize disease control [39]. Bone metastasis is a common site of disease in prostate cancer and is associated with skeletal-related events. Identifying patients with bone-dominant disease through bone imaging can guide the use of therapies targeting bone metastases, such as radiopharmaceuticals, radium^{223} [40]. 68Gallium-Prostate-Specific Membrane Antigen-11 (68Ga-PSMA-11) or 18Fluorine-DCFPyL (18F-DCFPyL) positron emission tomography (PET) scan imaging can identify patients with mCRPC who are suitable candidates for PSMA-targeted therapies like Pluvicto (lutetium Lu 177 vipivotide tetraxetan) [41]. Finally, D-dimer, Fibrinogen, and Platelet Levels are essential for monitoring the severity of DIC and assessing the risk of bleeding versus thrombosis. By leveraging these biomarkers, clinicians can tailor treatment strategies to the individual patient's tumor biology and clinical status, optimizing outcomes even in the face of complex and challenging conditions like DIC (**Figure 1**) [42, 43].

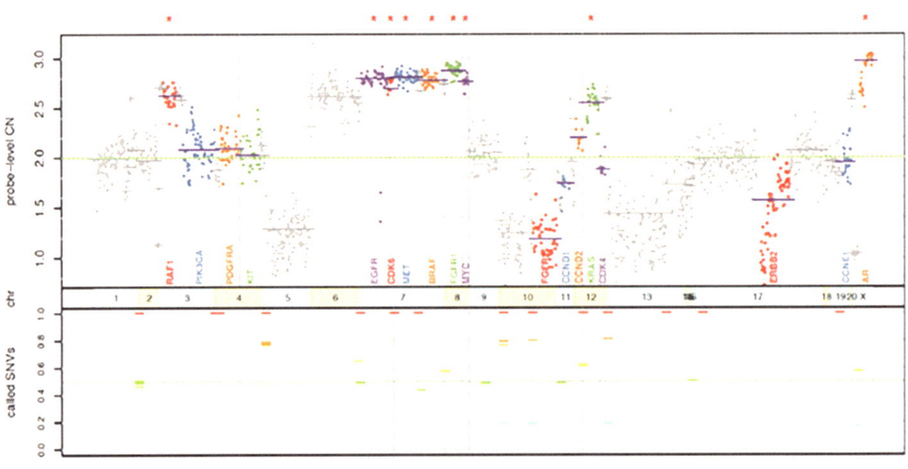

Figure 1.
The plot illustrates the gene amplification (*) of the androgen receptor (AR) gene and multiple tyrosine kinase receptor genes in a 68-Year-Old Patient with advanced Prostate Cancer at the time of onset of DIC. This patient, who had previously undergone extensive treatment for advanced prostate cancer, developed DIC, and ctDNA analysis revealed these genetic amplifications, which were not present at the time of diagnosis. The findings suggest a potential link between cancer progression, key oncogenic alterations, and the development of DIC. The patient was subsequently treated with mitoxantrone in combination with prednisone, leading to the resolution of DIC.

DOI: http://dx.doi.org/10.5772/intechopen.1008297

9. Conclusion

DIC associated with prostate cancer represents a rare but devastating complication that can occur in advanced prostate cancer, presenting significant challenges in diagnosis and clinical management. Despite its severity, DIC in prostate cancer remains an area with no specific guidelines or prospective trials to guide treatment. The management of DIC in the context of prostate cancer requires a multidisciplinary approach, including better understanding the underlying mechanisms, improving early diagnosis, and addressing both the underlying malignancy and the coagulation disorder. As our understanding of the molecular underpinnings of DIC in cancer evolves, new diagnostic tools and therapeutic strategies are likely to emerge. By tailoring treatment to the individual patient's clinical, genetic and molecular profile, clinicians can more effectively manage the complex interplay between cancer and coagulation, potentially improving outcomes and quality of life for patients facing this challenging condition.

Author details

William Schwartzman, Parker Wilson, Zane Gray and Jue Wang*
Department of Internal Medicine, Simmons Comprehensive Cancer Center,
UT Southwestern Medical Center, USA

*Address all correspondence to: jue.wang@utsouthwestern.edu

References

[1] Siegel RL, Giaquinto AN, Jemal A. Cancer statistics, 2024. CA: a Cancer Journal for Clinicians. 2024;**74**(1):12-49

[2] Schaeffer EM, Srinivas S, Adra N, et al. Prostate cancer, version 4.2023, NCCN clinical practice guidelines in oncology. Journal of the National Comprehensive Cancer Network : JNCCN. 2023;**21**(10):1067-1096

[3] Feinstein DI. Disseminated intravascular coagulation in patients with solid tumors. Oncology (Williston Park). 2015;**29**(2):96-102

[4] Hyman DM, Soff GA, Kampel LJ. Disseminated intravascular coagulation with excessive fibrinolysis in prostate cancer: A case series and review of the literature. Oncology. 2011;**81**(2):119-125

[5] Wang T et al. Amplification of multiple receptor tyrosine kinase pathways in a patient with metastatic castration-resistant prostate cancer with disseminated intravascular coagulation (DIC) ARC. Journal of Hematology. 2017;**2**(1):16-22

[6] Ni B, Wang J. Disseminated intravascular coagulation secondary to advanced prostate cancer: Clinical characteristics, management, and prognosis. Journal of Clinical Oncology. 2018;**36**(6_suppl):355-355. DOI: 10.1200/JCO.2018.36.6_suppl.355

[7] Tesselaar M et al. Microparticle-associated tissue factor activity: A link between cancer and thrombosis? Journal of Thrombosis and Haemostasis. 2007;**5**(3):520-527

[8] Hell L et al. Extracellular vesicle-associated tissue factor activity in prostate cancer patients with disseminated intravascular coagulation. Cancers. 2021;**13**(7):1487

[9] Fainchtein K, Tera Y, Kearn N, Noureldin A, Othman M. Hypercoagulability and thrombosis risk in prostate cancer: The Role of thromboelastography. Semin Thromb Hemost. 2023;**49**(2):111-118. DOI: 10.1055/s-0042-1758116

[10] Al Saleh HA et al. Thrombotic characteristics of extracellular vesicles derived from prostate cancer cells. The Prostate. 2018;**78**(13):953-961

[11] Navarro M et al. Patient with disseminated intravascular coagulation as the first manifestation of adenocarcinoma of the prostate. Risks of prostatic biopsy. Prostate Cancer and Prostatic Diseases. 2006;**9**(2):190-191

[12] Kohli M et al. Advanced prostate cancer activates coagulation: A controlled study of activation markers of coagulation in ambulatory patients with localized and advanced prostate cancer. Blood Coagulation & Fibrinolysis. 2002;**13**(1):1-5

[13] Nickel KF et al. The polyphosphate–factor XII pathway drives coagulation in prostate cancer-associated thrombosis. Blood, The Journal of the American Society of Hematology. 2015;**126**(11):1379-1389

[14] Ong SY, Taverna J, Jokerst C, Enzler T, Hammode E, Rogowitz E, et al. Prostate cancer-associated disseminated intravascular coagulation with excessive fibrinolysis treated with degarelix. Case Reports in Oncological Medicine. 2015;**2015**:212543

[15] Wada T, Gando S. Phenotypes of disseminated intravascular

coagulation. Thrombosis and Haemostasis. 2024;**124**(3):181-191. DOI: 10.1055/a-2165-1142

[16] Takada E et al. Intramuscular bleeding triggered by disseminated intravascular coagulation with enhanced fibrinolysis in a patient with prostate cancer. Internal Medicine. 2022;**61**(9):1411-1413

[17] Levi M. Disseminated intravascular coagulation in cancer: An update. Seminars in Thrombosis and Hemostasis. Jun 2019;**45**(4):342-347. DOI: 10.1055/s-0039-1687890

[18] Levi M et al. Guidelines for the diagnosis and management of disseminated intravascular coagulation. British Journal of Haematology. 2009;**145**(1):24-33

[19] Duran I, Tannock IF. Disseminated intravascular coagulation as the presenting sign of metastatic prostate cancer. Journal of General Internal Medicine. 2006;**21**(11):C6-C8

[20] Talebi TN, Manoharan M, Singal R. Resolution of thrombocytopenia secondary to disseminated intravascular coagulation with docetaxel chemotherapy in prostate cancer. American Journal of Therapeutics. 2012;**19**(1):e59-e61

[21] Gauthier H et al. Very fast recovery of acute disseminated intravascular coagulation with abiraterone acetate in a patient with bone metastases from castrate-resistant prostate cancer. Case Reports in Oncology. 2014;7(3):625-627

[22] Ruffion A et al. Successful use of samarium 153 for emergency treatment of disseminated intravascular coagulation due to metastatic hormone refractory prostate cancer. The Journal of Urology. 2000;**164**(3 Part 1):782-782

[23] Virgo KS, Rumble RB, Talcott J. Initial management of noncastrate advanced, recurrent, or metastatic prostate cancer: ASCO guideline update. Journal of Clinical Oncology. 2023;**41**(20):3652-3656

[24] Levi M, Scully M. How I treat disseminated intravascular coagulation. Blood, The Journal of the American Society of Hematology. 2018;**131**(8):845-854

[25] Squizzato A et al. Supportive management strategies for disseminated intravascular coagulation. Thrombosis and Haemostasis. 2016;**116**(05):896-904

[26] Rubin RN, Colman RW. Disseminated intravascular coagulation: Approach to treatment. Drugs. 1992;**44**(6):963-971

[27] Garnier D et al. Genetic pathways linking hemostasis and cancer. Thrombosis Research. 2012;**129**:S22-S29

[28] Boccaccio C, Medico E. Cancer and blood coagulation. Cellular and Molecular Life Sciences CMLS. 2006;**63**:1024-1027

[29] Tawil N, Bassawon R, Rak J. Oncogenes and clotting factors: The emerging role of tumor cell genome and epigenome in cancer-associated thrombosis. Seminars in Thrombosis and Hemostasis. 2019;**45**(4):373-384. DOI: 10.1055/s-0039-1687891

[30] Lee AY. Cancer and thromboembolic disease: Pathogenic mechanisms. Cancer Treatment Reviews. 2002;**28**(3):137-140

[31] Levi M. Cancer-related coagulopathies. Thrombosis Research. 2014;**133**(Suppl 2):S70-S75

[32] Boccaccio C, Comoglio PM. Genetic link between cancer and

thrombosis. Journal of Clinical Oncology. 2009;**27**(29):4827-4833

[33] D'Asti E, Rak J. Biological basis of personalized anticoagulation in cancer: Oncogene and oncomir networks as putative regulators of coagulopathy. Thrombosis Research. 2016;**140**:S37-S43

[34] Rak J, Klement P, Yu J. Genetic determinants of cancer coagulopathy, angiogenesis and disease progression. Vnitrni lekarstvi. 2006;**52**:135-138

[35] Ryan CJ, Tindall DJ. Androgen receptor rediscovered: The new biology and targeting the androgen receptor therapeutically. Journal of Clinical Oncology. 2011;**29**(27):3651-3658

[36] Hamid AA et al. Compound genomic alterations of TP53, PTEN, and RB1 tumor suppressors in localized and metastatic prostate cancer. European Urology. 2019;**76**(1):89-97

[37] de Bono J et al. Olaparib for metastatic castration-resistant prostate cancer. New England Journal of Medicine. 2020;**382**(22):2091-2102

[38] Le DT et al. PD-1 blockade in tumors with mismatch-repair deficiency. New England Journal of Medicine. 2015;**372**(26):2509-2520

[39] Schaeffer EM et al. Prostate cancer, version 4.2023, NCCN clinical practice guidelines in oncology. Journal of the National Comprehensive Cancer Network. 2023;**21**(10):1067-1096

[40] Parker C et al. Alpha emitter radium-223 and survival in metastatic prostate cancer. New England Journal of Medicine. 2013;**369**(3):213-223

[41] Sartor O et al. Lutetium-177–PSMA-617 for metastatic castration-resistant prostate cancer. New England Journal of Medicine. 2021;**385**(12):1091-1103

[42] Wang J. Applying precision medicine approach to metastatic castration-resistant prostate cancer: Urgent education needs on genomic oncology. Journal of Molecular Oncology Research. 2017;**1**(2):79-83

[43] Wang TR, Ding ZH, Boddupalli S, Wong D, Wang J. Overcoming chemotherapy resistance by targeting IGF-1 axis in a patient with metastatic castration-resistant prostate cancer: Killing two birds with one stone. Journal of Clinical Research and Case Studies. 2017;**2**(2):70-74

Chapter 6

Endovascular Techniques for the Treatment of Venous Diseases

Leonardo da Cruz Renó
and Angélica Araújo Cortines Laxe Renó

Abstract

This chapter analyzes the use of minimally invasive endovascular techniques for the treatment of acute and chronic venous diseases, demonstrating their improved use due to the development of new materials and improved techniques. We conclude that today, we can treat everything from acute venous thrombosis, with the aim of reducing progression to chronic venous disease, to pulmonary embolism, with the aim of reducing mortality and improving quality of life. In addition, pulmonary embolism is prevented with vena cava filters that are increasingly easy to implant, and venous compressions and chronic venous occlusions are treated with stents dedicated to the venous system.

Keywords: venous thrombosis, thromboembolic disease, pulmonary embolism, vena cava filters, venous insufficiency

1. Introduction

Venous thromboembolism (VTE), including deep vein thrombosis (DVT) and pulmonary embolism (PE), is the third most common cardiovascular condition after myocardial infarction and stroke, with an estimated incidence between 0.7 and 2 per 1000 person-years [1]. Patients typically develop venous thromboembolism because of any modifications associated with the classic Virchow triad (**Figure 1**), which delineates the underlying physiological changes that precipitate the formation of thrombi within the venous system. These alterations encompass those affecting the venous wall, the process of blood coagulation, and the characteristics of blood flow [2].

Chronic obstruction is the predominant aspect in approximately one-third of patients with post-thrombotic syndrome (PTS), in addition to valve reflux and varicose veins [3].

Up to 50% of patients with DVT will develop PTS within 2 years, with 10% of those cases being the most severe. Patients with iliofemoral DVT are at a higher risk of developing PTS (70–80%) [4]. Obstruction in the iliac-femoral segment, with or without reflux leads to high levels of venous hypertension (**Figure 2**). Therefore, a more aggressive approach is recommended in the acute phase of this type of proximal DVT, as recanalization rates are low (20–30%) by anticoagulation therapy alone

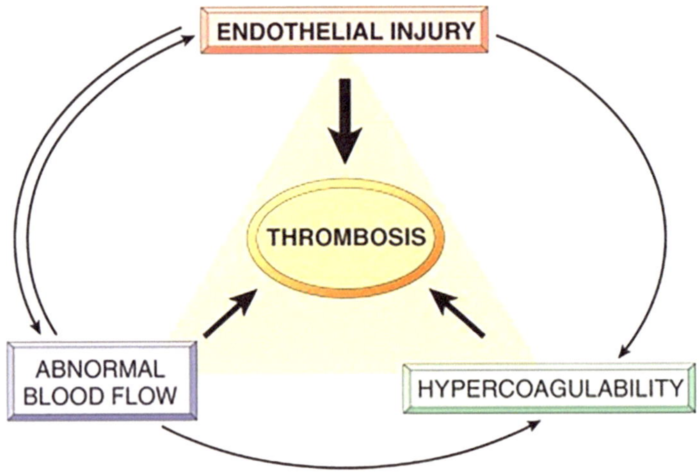

Figure 1.
Virchow Triad scheme. Available from: https://www.medicinehack.com/2011/07/virchows-triad.html

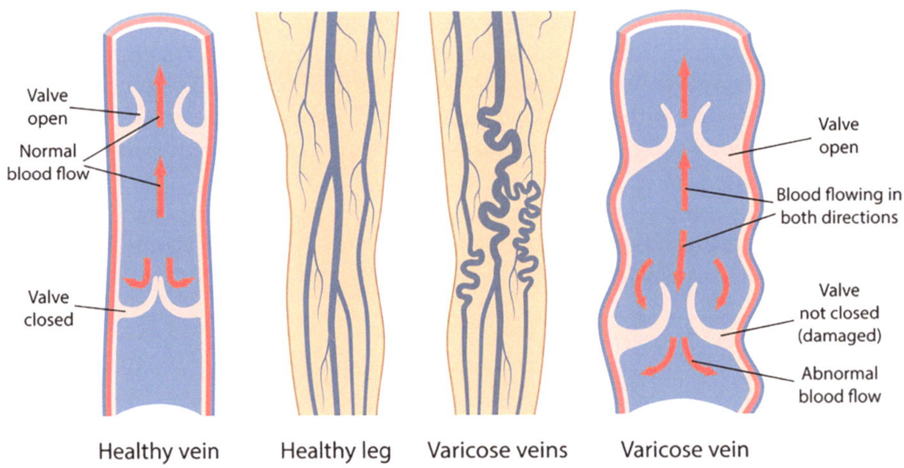

Figure 2.
Scheme of venous valve dysfunction. Available from: www.veinstreatment.com

is used, especially in younger patients [5]. Chronic venous obstruction: diagnostic considerations and therapeutic role of percutaneous iliac stenting [6].

Therefore, if possible, iliofemoral DVT should be treated in the acute phase with thrombolysis/thrombectomy to prevent the high morbidity associated with PTS. As a result, some of these patients will need to be treated in the chronic phase. However, many patients have contraindications to the use of anticoagulants or thrombolytics, and in these cases, the use of vena cava filters and compression stocking may be the one treatment possible [7, 8].

The development of endovascular procedures has revolutionized the diagnosis and treatment of chronic venous obstruction. In 2000, Neglén and Raju published a major case series on the technical aspects and initial clinical outcomes of angioplasty with auto-expandable stents. They achieved a technical success rate of 98% and primary patency rates of 82, 91 (assisted primary), and 92% (secondary) for 1 year.

Although multicenter randomized studies have not been published, the literature suggests recommendations with level 1B evidence due to the low risk of the procedure compared to the benefits. This is especially true for patients with disabling symptoms where clinical treatment is ineffective and conventional Palma surgery or prosthesis is the only available option [9, 10].

Pulmonary embolism is a potentially fatal complication of DVT, with an annual incidence rate of VTE ranging between 75 and 269 cases per 100,000 persons [11, 12]. It has an acute phase with high morbimortality and a chronic phase, when the patient should develop sequels, like pulmonary hypertension and right cardiac failure [13]. The development of the tomographic images with contrast allows an accurate diagnosis in emergency settings, and the novel oral anticoagulants show very safe and effective treatment to many patients. In the PE with right cardiac stress and elevated levels of cardiac biomarkers, today have devices to allow a quick cleaning of pulmonary tree [14].

Finishing the chapter, we discuss the vena cava filters, an important device to avoid mortality by PE in patients with high risk of DVT or with DVT but contraindications to anticoagulants [15]. The chapter highlights the three main factors that contribute to venous congestion and hypertension: reflux caused by valve incompetence, obstruction of venous drainage, weakness in the calf muscle pump, and other complications like pulmonary embolism (PE) and these treatments.

2. Pulmonary embolism

PE is the leading cause of preventable death in hospitalized patients [16]. Around 40–60% of symptomatic DVT cases have asymptomatic venous thromboembolism (EP), and 50–70% of symptomatic EP cases have asymptomatic DVT. It is estimated that around 600,000 cases of PE occur in the United States each year, with a mortality rate of around 300,000. Acute PE is the third leading cause of death in hospitalized patients [17].

It is thought that there are three basic categories of acute PE: simple PE, without hypotension or signs of right heart overload; sub-massive PE, with signs of right ventricular overload but without hypotension; and massive PTE, with hypotension and signs of severe right ventricular overload [18].

The pathophysiology of PE is characterized by the direct physical obstruction of the pulmonary arteries, hypoxic vasoconstriction, and the release of potent pulmonary arterial vasoconstrictors, which further increase pulmonary vascular resistance and right ventricular afterload. Acute pressure overload of the right ventricle can result in hypokinesia and dilatation of the right ventricle, tricuspid regurgitation, and associated insufficiency. A significant overload of the right ventricle can result in increased exertion, which may lead to ischemia due to increased myocardial oxygen demand and concomitant limitations of its supply due to hypoxemia and increased parietal tension [19, 20].

2.1 Percutaneous intervention indications

In the event of an acute PTE, it is imperative that risk stratification be conducted expeditiously, with the optimal intervention then being implemented. The management of pulmonary embolism (PE) has become more complex due to the expanded role of catheter-based therapies, surgical thrombectomies, and cardiac assist technologies, such as right ventricular assistance devices and extracorporeal support. The heterogeneous nature of PE necessitates a multidisciplinary team approach [21, 22].

The American College of Chest Physicians (ACCP) has recommended that percutaneous catheter-directed therapy (CDT) be considered in patients with pulmonary thromboembolism (PE) associated with hypotension and who have contraindications to systemic thrombolysis, unsuccessful thrombolysis, or shock [23].

Currently, computer tomography (CT) angiography represents the most effective diagnostic and assessment tool for identifying the anatomical severity of PE [24]. However, it is not without limitations, including cost, availability, and the use of high volumes of contrast. In instances where the use of contrast is not desired, transthoracic echocardiography can be employed to assess the hemodynamic consequences of PE and indicate the necessity for more invasive intervention. Additionally, bedside intravascular ultrasound can be utilized to identify central pulmonary emboli [25].

The identification of right ventricular overload allows for the stratification of risk in normotensive patients with PE, indicating the potential for treatment other than anticoagulation [26]. Echocardiographic findings indicative of the condition include hypokinesia and dilatation of the right ventricle, flattening of the interventricular septum and paradoxical movement toward the left ventricle, as well as an abnormal trans mitral Doppler flow profile, tricuspid regurgitation, pulmonary hypertension with a maximum tricuspid jet velocity greater than 2.6 m/sec, and loss of inspiratory collapse of the inferior vena cava. A ratio of the diameter of the right ventricle to that of the left ventricle (RV/LV) greater than 0.9, as assessed by transthoracic echocardiography in the left parasternal and subcostal axes, has been identified as an independent predictor of hospital mortality (**Figure 3**). Another piece of data

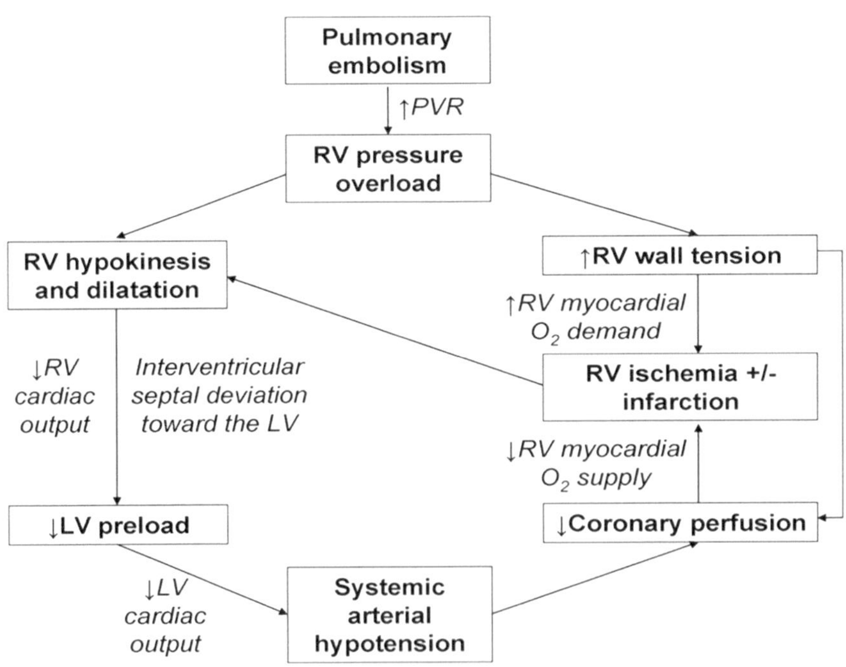

Figure 3.
The pathophysiology of acute PE. PVR indicates pulmonary vascular resistance. (Reprinted with permission from: Ref. [27]).

to be analyzed is the size of the right ventricle in relation to the left ventricle on CT. The same cut-off of 0.9 predicts sub-massive PE and predicts higher morbidity and mortality with a greater chance of long-term sequelae in surviving cases [28, 29].

Moreover, in patients with pulmonary embolism and contraindications to thrombolytic and anticoagulant therapy, the implantation of an inferior vena cava filter should be considered. Endovascular management of pulmonary embolism can be divided into two categories: therapeutic and prophylactic treatments. Prophylactic treatment includes the placement of an inferior vena cava filter, whereas endovascular therapeutic interventions encompass a range of catheter-directed therapies. The indications for both modalities have evolved over the past decade in response to the emergence of new evidence [30].

2.2 Percutaneous endovascular techniques

Catheter-directed thrombolysis (CDT) for pulmonary thromboembolism (PE) is carried out using low-profile catheters and devices, mechanical embolus, and thrombus fragmentation and/or catheter-directed embolus aspiration, with or without intrathrombus thrombolytic injection. The decision as to whether thrombolytics are used in CDT and their dose will depend on the expected risk of bleeding. The ultimate objective is to reduce the central thrombus, thereby alleviating the cardiac overload that is the underlying cause of death and improving pulmonary and systemic oxygenation. In the case of massive PE, catheter-directed thrombolysis with associated mechanical methods is carried out, while in sub-massive PTE, only catheterization and intrathrombus infusion of thrombolytics can be performed [31, 32].

2.3 Catheter-directed thrombolysis

The rationale for catheter-directed thrombolysis (CDT), which was established in patients with acute arterial occlusion, is that rapid lysis is achieved with lower doses of thrombolytic therapy, resulting in fewer serious bleeding complications. Interventional catheterization techniques for massive pulmonary embolism (PE) include mechanical fragmentation of thrombus with a standard pulmonary artery catheter, clot pulverization with a rotating basket catheter, percutaneous rheolytic thrombectomy, or pigtail rotational catheter embolectomy. If the risk of bleeding is not significant, it is possible to combine pharmacologic thrombolysis and mechanical interventions [33].

The objective of catheter extraction of thrombus is to reduce pulmonary arterial resistance to a sufficient extent to alleviate pulmonary artery hypertension, thereby alleviating right ventricular dilatation and dysfunction and rapidly increasing cardiac output. Catheter embolectomy rarely results in the extraction of massive pulmonary arterial thrombus. Instead, more often, clot fragments are suctioned through the catheter or displaced distally, resulting in only modest angiographic improvement [34].

In accordance with the contemporary definition of CDT, two principal protocols may be employed. In the case of massive PE, the catheter-directed thrombolytic drug bolus is utilized in conjunction with mechanical clot fragmentation and/or aspiration, with the objective of rapidly reducing the central clot. Flow studies have demonstrated the significant importance of fragmenting the thrombus and directing the infusion into the thrombus to achieve greater effectiveness in dissolving the thrombus [35].

3. Acute DVT

Thromboembolic disease is a multifactorial disorder with a prevalence ranging from 0.9 to 1.84/100,000 people/year. In acute cases, the most feared condition is pulmonary embolism (PE). DVT can be proximal or distal [36]. Only about 50 percent of patients with DVT have obvious clinical signs and symptoms, so scores have been developed to define the likelihood of testing for the condition, with the Wells score being the most widely used. The most commonly performed initial test for suspected cases is venous color Doppler ultrasound [37]. The clinical diagnosis of DVT is imprecise because only 20 to 40 percent of patients with symptoms are confirmed by symptoms are confirmed by objective tests. On the other hand, 15 to 50 percent of DVT cases do not present a DVT with a characteristic initial clinical picture. Therefore, the definitive diagnosis is based on complementary investigations. Among the available diagnostic methods, Duplex Mapping (DM) is considered the gold standard in non-invasive tests, showing good sensitivity and specificity for proximal and specificity for proximal DVT. However, this accuracy decreases for distal DVT (in the leg veins), with sensitivity and specificity of around 70 in this segment [38]. The risk of pulmonary embolism appears to be low in isolated DVT of the leg veins, but there is a risk of progression of distal thrombosis to proximal segments to proximal segments of up to 20%. For this reason, some authors believe that in cases of negative MD for DVT, it should be repeated within 7 days to detect thrombi in days to detect thrombi in progression. To simplify the diagnostic approach, [39] Wells et al. developed a clinical prediction model that model that classifies patients according to their risk of DVT. This model, combined with non-invasive complementary tests, has been shown in several studies in the diagnosis of DVT [40].

Also, acute deep vein thrombosis can develop in addition to PE, phlegmasia cerulea dolens, or phlegmasia alba dolens (**Table 1**).

- Plegmasia cerulea dolens is a rare complication of DVT, usually due to extensive iliofemoral DVT [41]. It is a medical emergency requiring immediate treatment with a risk of death and limb loss. Secondary involvement of the arterial system may occur [42]. Clinically, there is significant asymmetric edema, pain, and compartment syndrome with the absence of distal pulses and neurological symptoms. Cancer, hypercoagulable states, vena cava filters, previous

Clinical characteristics	Score
Current Câncer	1
Paresy, paralisy, immobilization	1
Immobilization >3 days or major surgery until 4 weeks	1
Sensibility in deeper veins	1
Calf swelling >3 cm	
Depressible swelling	
Superficial colateral veins	
Other probabli diagnosys	

Table 1.
Wells score for DVT.

PTV, oral contraceptives, venous stasis, and trauma are the most common risk factors [43]. It can range from uncomplicated PCD to venous gangrene and, if not treated in time, has an amputation rate of 12–25% and a mortality rate of 25–40% [44].

In the case of compartment syndrome, fasciotomy should be performed prior to any intervention. Venous release should then be attempted [45].

In this case study, a 45-year-old male patient with no additional medical conditions was admitted to the emergency department with a sudden onset of pain in his left lower limb. Upon physical examination, we observed stiffness of the entire limb and severe cyanosis. He was immediately submitted to decompressive fasciotomy of the thigh and leg, with indication for mechanical thrombolysis with a rheolytic device the following day, as the images below show. This procedure required the use of a stent in the left iliac artery and implantation of a vena cava filter beforehand. There was no evidence of thrombophilia or neoplasia, only evidence of previous mechanical obstruction of the common iliac left vein (**Figures 4–12**).

Pharmacomechanical thrombectomy has the same final outcomes in cases of phlegmasia cerulea and alba dolens as catheter-directed thrombolysis, but the treatment time is shorter, and there is a potential reduction in the dose of fibrinolytic used. There are also reports of a lower chance of developing post-thrombotic syndrome when using rapid pharmacomechanical thrombolysis while preserving the venous valves [46].

Phlegmasia Alba Dolens – is another rare complication of iliofemoral DVT, usually with significant pain and swelling throughout the limb. There may be arterial vasospasm, coldness, and reduced pulses. Pulmonary embolism is more common in patients with proximal than distal DVT and occurs in more than 50% of proximal DVTs with a mortality rate of 5–30%. It may lead to rhabdomyolysis but less than phlegmasia cerulea dolens [44].

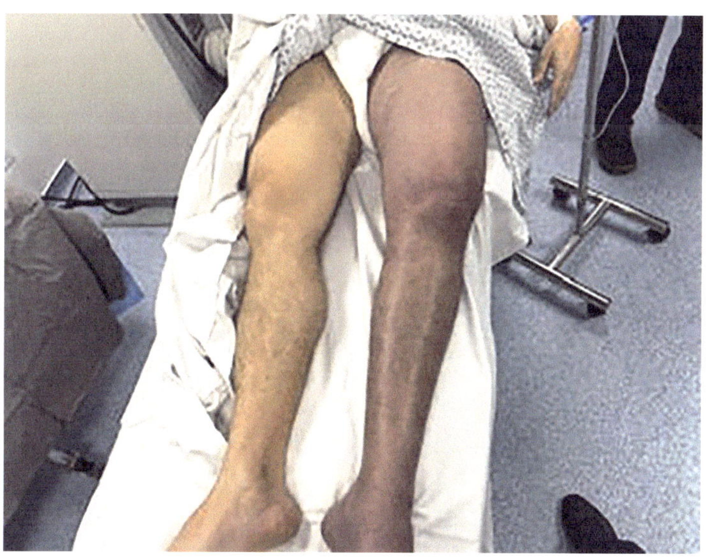

Figure 4.
Phelgmasia cerúlea dolens in left side.

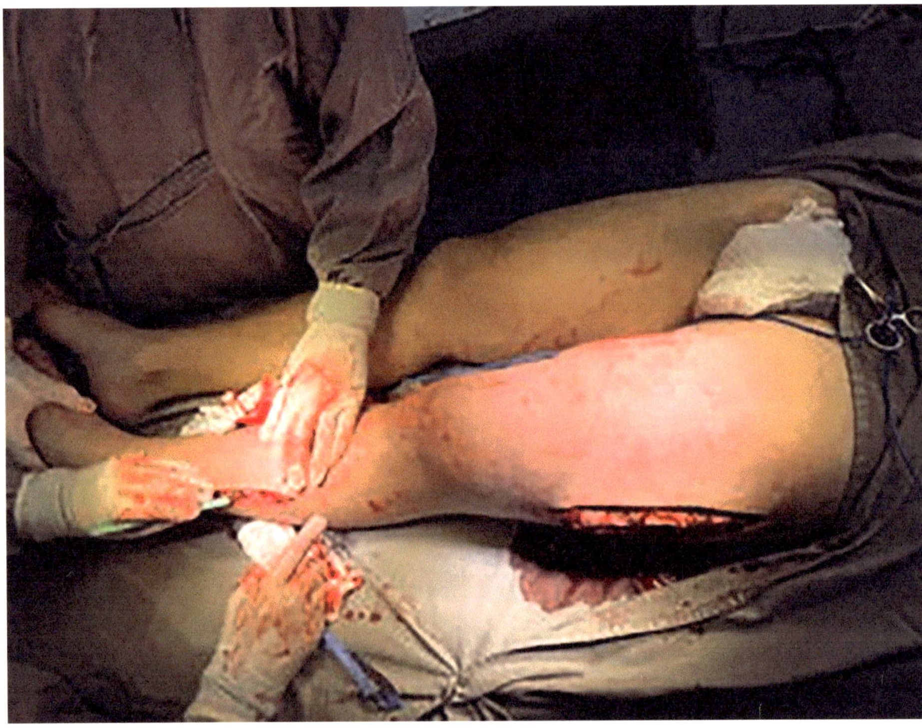

Figure 5.
Emergencial fasciotomy.

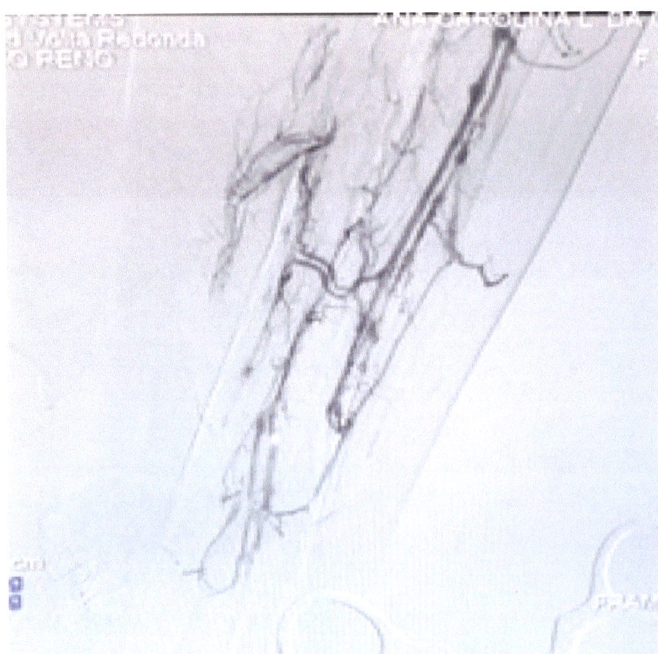

Figure 6.
Thrombosed leg veins visualized by distal venography with direct function.

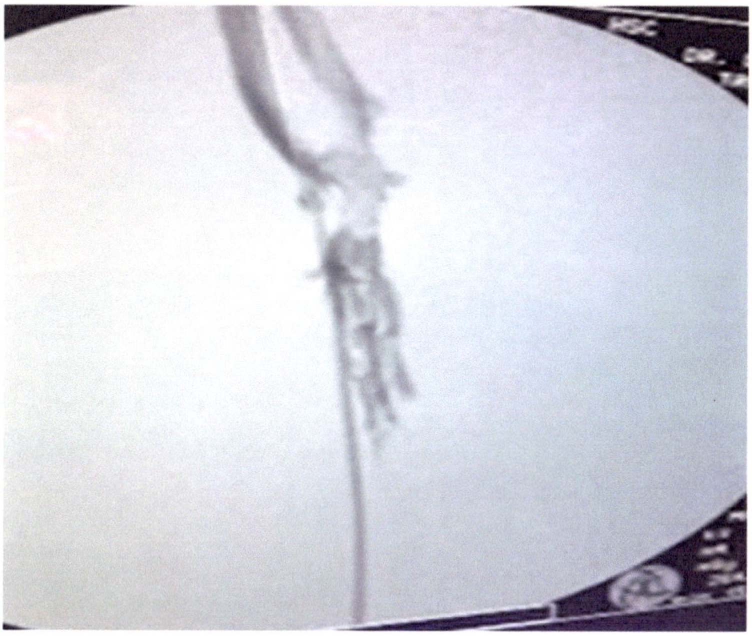

Figure 7.
Popliteal vein catheterization by open view of tibial vein distally.

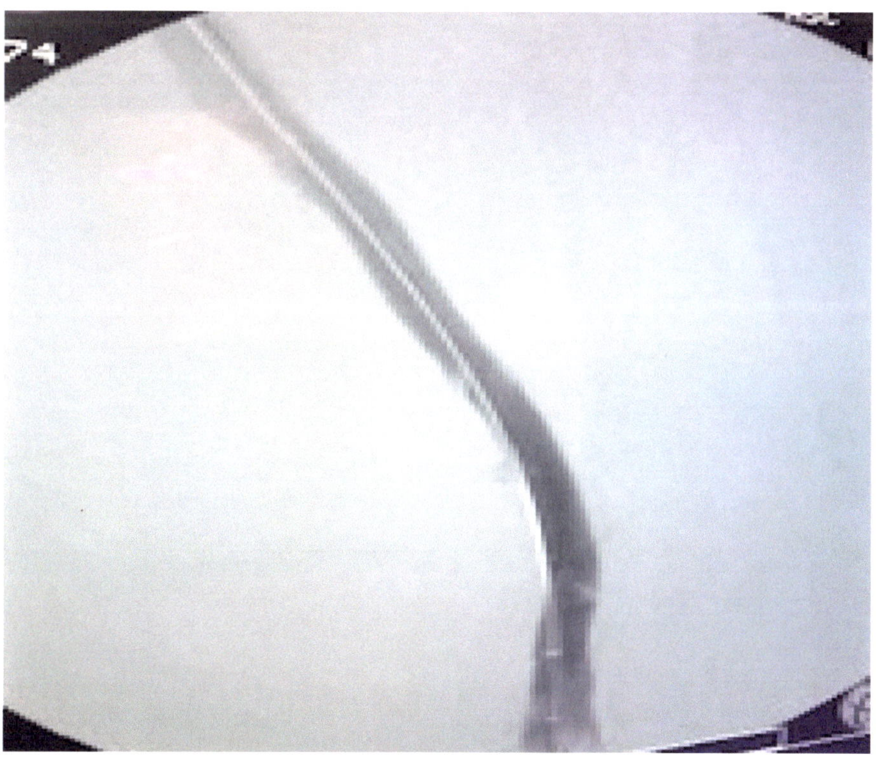

Figure 8.
Femoral vein after pharmacomechanical thrombolysis.

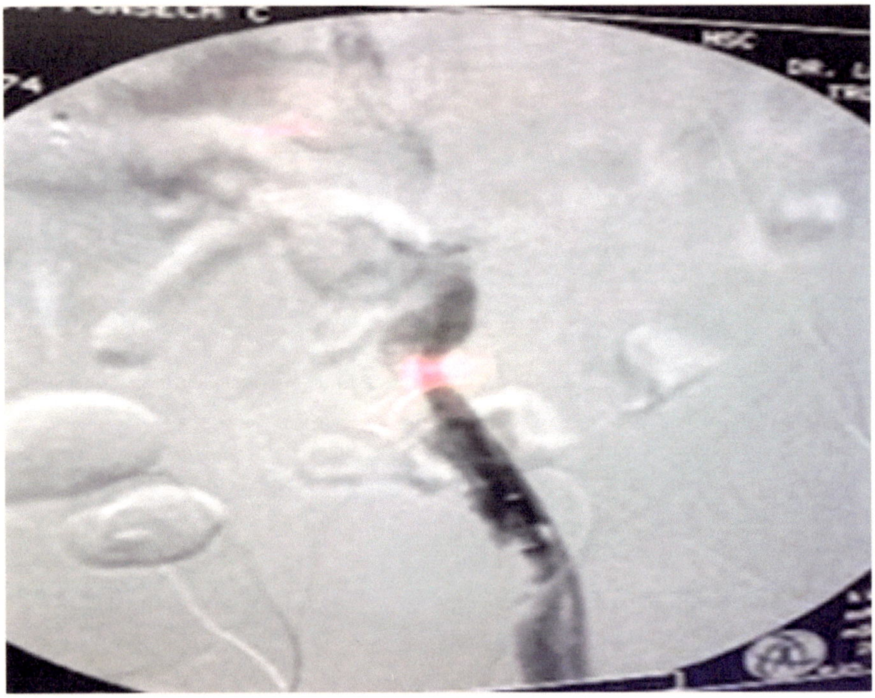

Figure 9.
Iliac vein obstruction.

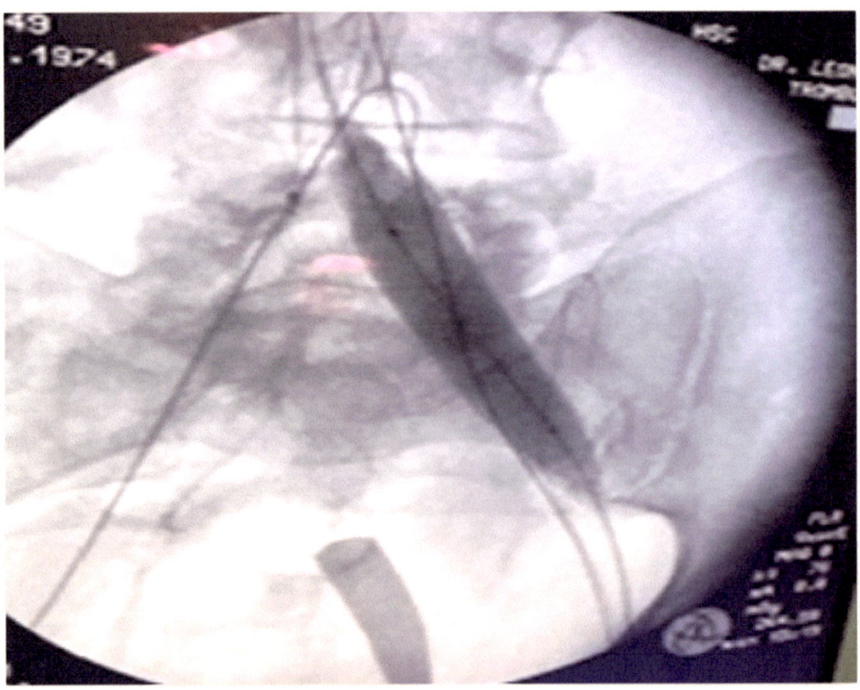

Figure 10.
Angioplasty with ballonn and stenting after reccanalization of occlusion.

DOI: http://dx.doi.org/10.5772/intechopen.1007880

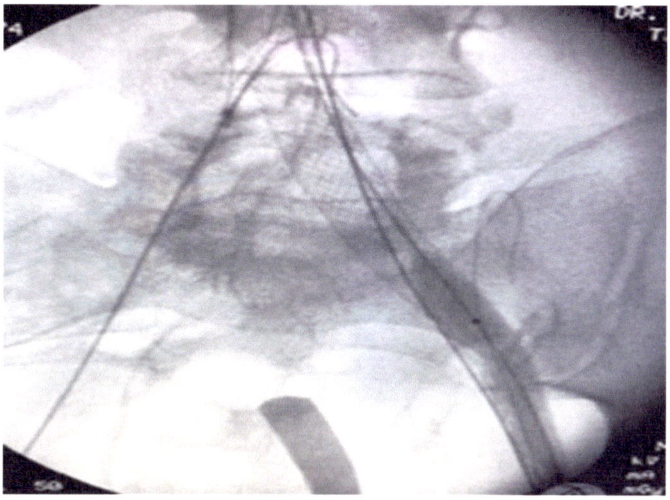

Figure 11.
Ballon angioplasty of external ilíaca left vein and stentitng.

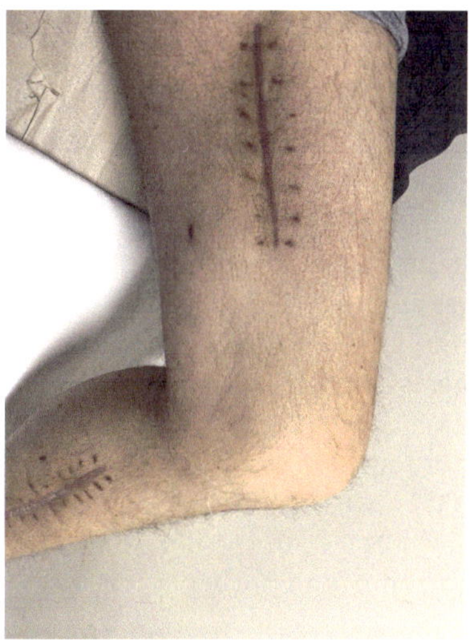

Figure 12.
Final aspect after 1 month in the same patient without any sequelae.

4. Chronic DVT

Following an acute DVT episode, if the patient does not develop a fatal pulmonary embolism and can undergo outpatient anticoagulant treatment, they may show significant improvement, with complete lysis of the thrombi and few sequelae o ris possible that varying degrees of intraluminal fibrosis may develop, which could potentially lead to some long-term consequences [47]. These could include persistent edema, venous claudication, leg ulcers, and a significant worsening of quality of life [48]. The most common treatment is the use of compression stockings, phlebotonics and physical exercise [49]. However, some cases do not respond to these measures, and endovascular treatment is indicated. In such cases, stents are more commonly used in iliac occlusions. PTS is a complication with a significant public health impact, with a range of signs and symptoms including chronic pain, edema, hyperpigmentation, and stasis ulcers in the lower limbs occurring approximately 2 years after the acute DVT episode [50].

Historically, the treatment of DVT has been based on full anticoagulation. However, even before the development of modern imaging techniques and endovascular surgery, attempts were made to improve the living conditions of severely symptomatic patients due to iliac obstructions. One such attempt was the classic Palma operation. However, due to their greater invasion and the need for experienced surgeons to achieve optimal outcomes, they are now performed with great infrequency, with angioplasty with stents becoming the preferred approach [51, 52].

5. Indications for endovascular treatment

Patients with previous non-rechanneled iliac-femoral DVT, venous claudication, volumous and refractory edema, ochre dermatitis, dermofibrosis, and stasis ulcers [53].

5.1 Examination

Venous duplex ultrasound plays an important role in the follow-up and diagnosis of patients with PTS, but it has shortcomings when it comes to examining the iliac veins, which are not well visualized by the method [54]. Other image evaluations are venous magnetic resonance angiography, a good option, especially in the iliac cava region and in cases where the use of iodinated contrast is contraindicated. It has limitations in terms of access and cost [55].

Peripheral vein intravenous (IV) contrast tomography is the most widely used test for preoperative diagnosis and surgical planning. In addition to providing images of the iliofemoral axis, it evaluates surrounding structures that may cause compression and other pathologies that may confuse the diagnosis. Venography by computer tomography (CT) angiography or direct venous angiography is a technique that has shown advantages in the detail of the images compared to the usual technique, since deep veins are poorly contrasted due to the travel time of the contrast agent [56].

This technique involves puncturing a vein in the foot and watching the contrast flow cranially. It is a better technique for assessing flow before surgery. Venography is an objective test and is still considered the gold standard for the assessment of chronic DVT. It is ideally performed by US-guided puncture [57].

Intravascular ultrasound (IVUS) has been recommended as the best diagnostic tool in iliofemoral disease, as it allows a better understanding of the etiology of the lesion, vessel diameter, and wall thickening and contributes to better accuracy of stent implantation [57, 58].

Testing for thrombophilia is important in cases of recurrent thrombosis, thrombosis with an unknown cause in young patients and those with a known family history of venous thromboembolism, as well as in rare cases such as splanchnic thrombosis, cerebral thrombosis and thrombosis resistant to anticoagulant therapy, and involves testing to antiphospholipid syndrome and the presence of lupus anticoagulants or anticardiolipin/anti-beta2 glycoprotein IgG or IgM [59].

5.2 Procedure

If the lesion is an isolated iliac lesion, single access can be made via the femoral common vein, but depending on the extent of the segment involved, punctures may be made in the popliteal vein in the prone position, the internal saphenous vein, the femoral vein in the thigh, the external saphenous vein, and the jugular vein.

After puncture, hydrophilic guidewires with a 0.035 angled tip, a 5fr introducer, and diagnostic catheters are used. Larger introducers up to 10 Fr are used for stent and balloon implantation. In terms of the angioplasty balloon used, the balloon catheter chosen should preferably be non-compliant to allow angioplasty at high pressure, and its size should be appropriate for the large diameter of the veins [60]. Today, we have other specific stents for the venous territory with good radial strength and flexibility [61].

Despite some differences, they should all have common characteristics such as larger sizes, greater resistance to extrinsic compression, and a balance between radial strength and flexibility.

The entire obstructed segment should be treated so that the inflow has an unobstructed passage to the outflow. In the case of veins, due to their high elasticity, stents should always be used, avoiding the primary balloon. An important consideration is the patency of the deep femoral vein and its outflow into the common femoral vein to maintain good inflow to the stent, especially if the femoral vein in the thigh is occluded [62, 63].

Following is a real-life case demonstration with a 24-year-old patient who presented with DVT after taking oral contraceptives. After 3 months of treatment with compression stockings and full anticoagulation with rivaroxaban, her condition did not improve, with edema, venous claudication, and cyanosis in the evening in the lower right limb. Venous Doppler ultrasound of the left lower limb was requested, revealing recanalization

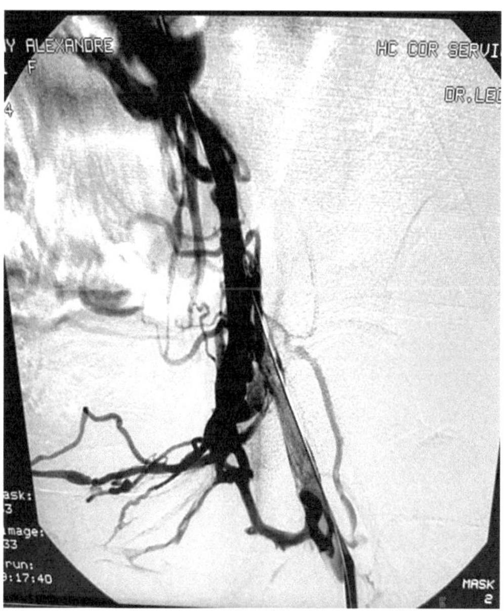

Figure 13.
Venography after ultrasound-guided puncture of the femoral vein in the thigh with fibrosis in the femoral veins and signs of chronic left iliac occlusion.

in the popliteal and femoral veins in the thigh and deep vein, but still with fibrosis and no recanalization in the common femoral and iliac veins. Angio tomography conformed to the picture, so we requested an endovascular procedure aimed at iliofemoral recanalization with a stent, as described below (**Figures 13–18**).

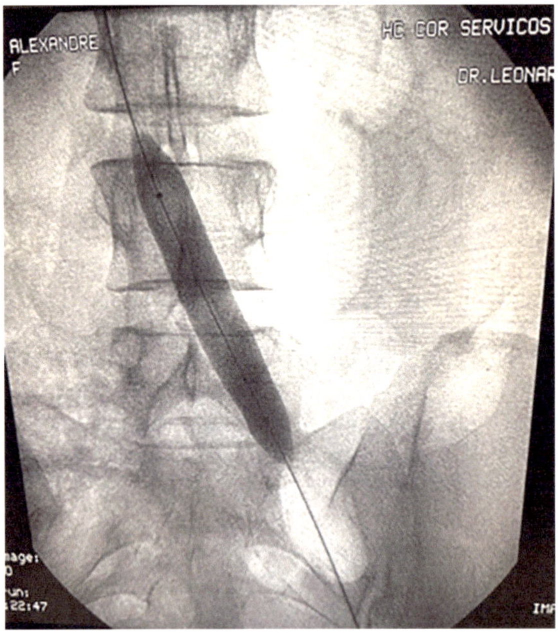

Figure 14.
After passing the hydrophilic stiff guidewire under the vert catheter, pre-dilation with a 4 mm × 100 balloon and then a 12 mm × 60 balloon.

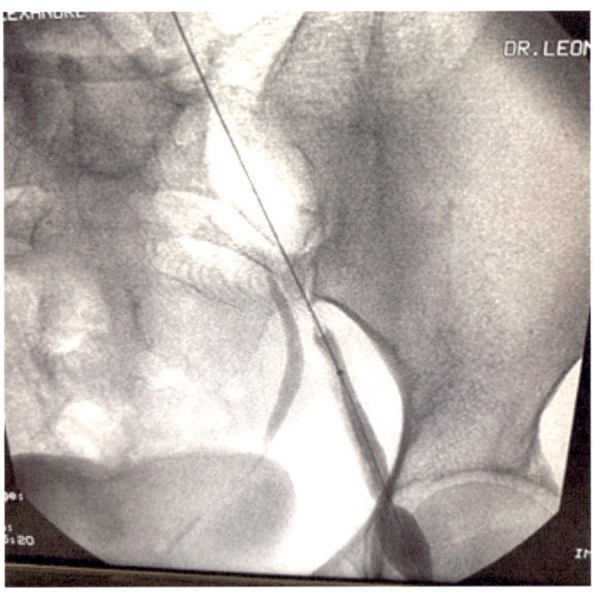

Figure 15.
Intense resistance to dilation by the balloon is observed due to fibrosis.

DOI: http://dx.doi.org/10.5772/intechopen.1007880

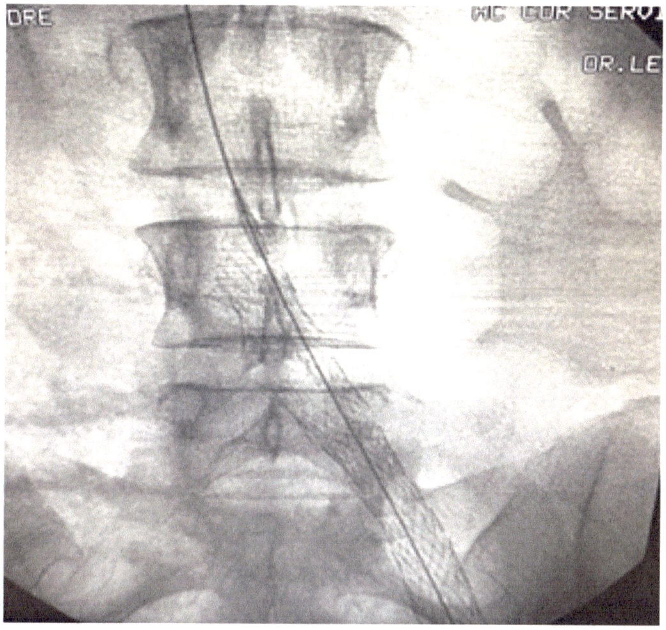

Figure 16.
After dilation, implantation of 16 × 150 and 14 × 100 dedicated venous Stents with an overlap area of 4 to 6 cm.

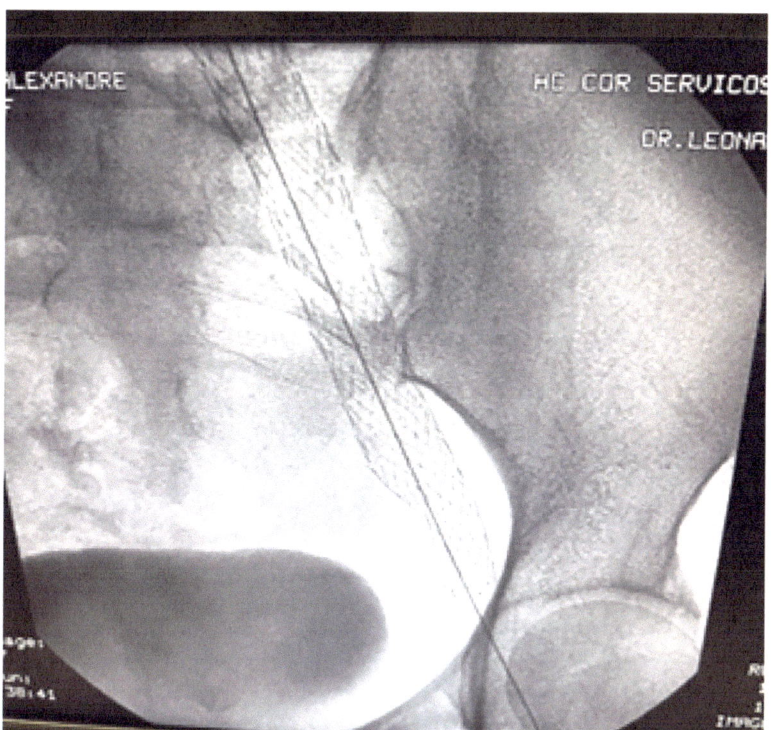

Figure 17.
The stents were extended to a healthy area of femoral inflow below the entrance to the deep femoral artery, which was patent.

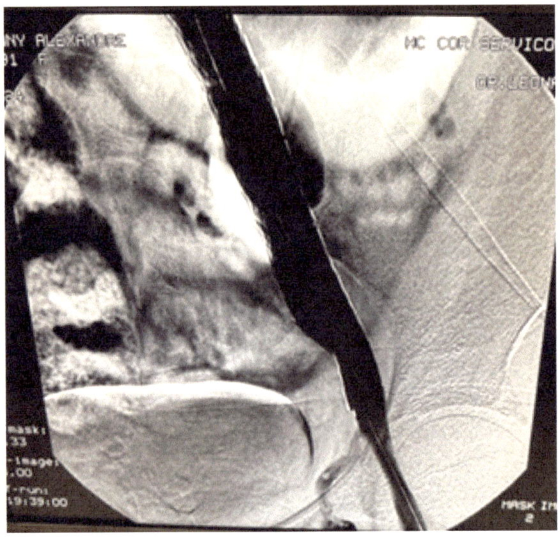

Figure 18.
Final appearance with good flow through the stents and absence of contrast in the collateral circulation.

6. Vena cava filters

Anticoagulant treatment is the standard and can prevent PE in cases of iliofemoral DVT in up to 95% of cases. However, there are situations where the use of anticoagulants is contraindicated or there is a risk of PE even when anticoagulation is prescribed. In such cases, the use of inferior vena cava filters is recommended [64].

The recurrence rate in properly treated patients is between 1.2 and 1.4%, and the incidence of recurrent and fatal PE is less than 0.1% [65].

Thrombi that embolize into the pulmonary artery mostly originates from the lower extremities. Therefore, methods have been developed over the years to obstruct the flow from the lower limbs to the pulmonary arteries to prevent pulmonary embolism. The initial procedure performed was the ligation of the inferior vena cava, which was carried out by Trendelenburg in 1906 [66].

The external clip placement in the inferior vena cava was first described in 1939. The Mobin-Uddin umbrella was the first filter created in the early 1970s [67, 68].

Technological advances have led to more effective devices with fewer complications and smaller calipers, even allowing bedside implantation using ultrasound [69].

The Kimray Greenfield filter was introduced shortly after the Mobin-Uddin filter. Its conical design and stainless-steel structure have since become the industry standard [70].

Clinical diagnosis of pulmonary embolism is challenging and often unreliable. The multicenter PIOPED study revealed no significant clinical differences between patients with confirmed pulmonary embolism and those without. Shockingly, only 30% of patients who died because of PE were correctly diagnosed, and between 30 and 50% of diagnostic angiographies performed yielded positive results [71].

CT angiography has a sensitivity of more than 90% for diagnosing pulmonary artery embolism, according to the PIOPED 2 study (**Figure 19**) [72].

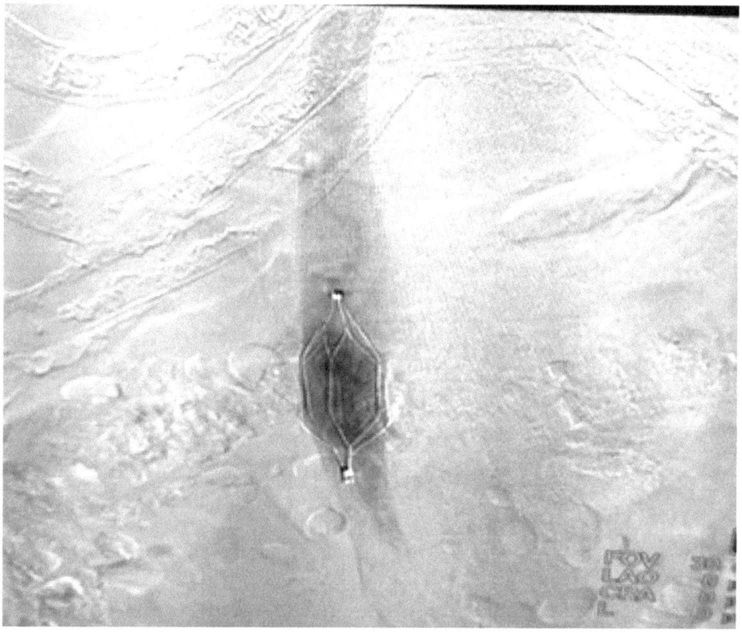

Figure 19.
Vena cava filter implanted in infrarenal position (author).

7. Conclusions

Endovascular surgery has demonstrated significant effectiveness and applicability in treating arterial, coronary, and cerebrovascular systems. Recently, new techniques and devices have expanded their use in treating venous diseases, resulting in more effective treatment and less morbidity in situations that previously required aggressive surgery, such as chronic venous obstructions and pulmonary thromboembolism.

Conflict of interest

The authors declare no conflict of interest.

Author details

Leonardo da Cruz Renó[1]* and Angélica Araújo Cortines Laxe Renó[2]

1 Unimed Hospital, Volta Redonda, Brazil

2 Hinja Hospital, Volta Redonda, Brazil

*Address all correspondence to: c.t.v.r@hotmail.com

References

[1] Anderson FA, Wheeler HB, Goldberg RJ, Hosmer DW, Patwardhan NA, Jovanovic B, et al. A population-based perspective of the hospital incidence and case-fatality rates of deep vein thrombosis and pulmonary embolism: The Worcester DVT study. Archives of Internal Medicine. 1991;**151**(5):933-938

[2] Brotman DJ, Deitcher SR, Lip GY, Matzdorff AC. Virchow's triad revisited. Southern Medical Journal. 2004;**97**(2):213-215

[3] Lee JJ, Al-Jubouri M, Acino R, Comerota AJ, Lurie F. Role of coexisting contralateral primary venous disease in development of post-thrombotic syndrome following catheter-based treatment of iliofemoral deep venous thrombosis. Journal of Vascular Surgery: Venous and Lymphatic Disorders. 2015;**3**(4):354-357. DOI: 10.1016/j.jvsv.2015.05.004. ISSN 2213-333X

[4] Prandoni P, Kahn SR. Post-thrombotic syndrome: Prevalence, prognostication and need for progress. British Journal of Haematology. 2009;**145**(3):286-295

[5] Raju S, Neglén P. Percutaneous recanalization of total occlusions of the iliac vein. Journal of Vascular Surgery. 2009;**50**(2):360-368

[6] Neglén P, Hollis KC, Olivier J, Raju S. Stenting of the venous outflow in chronic venous disease: Long-term stent-related outcome, clinical, and hemodynamic result. Journal of Vascular Surgery. 2007;**46**(5):979-990

[7] O'Sullivan GJ, Semba CP, Bittner CA, Kee ST, Razavi MK, Sze DY, et al. Endovascular management of iliac vein compression (May-Thurner) syndrome. Journal of Vascular and Interventional Radiology. 2000;**11**(7):823-836

[8] Raju S. Best management options for chronic iliac vein stenosis and occlusion. Journal of Vascular Surgery. 2013;**57**(4):1163-1169

[9] Jayaraj A, Meissner M. Impact of graduated compression stockings on the prevention of post-thrombotic syndrome-results of a randomized controlled trial. Phlebology. 2015;**30**(8):541-548

[10] Neglén P, Raju S. Balloon dilation and stenting of chronic iliac vein obstruction: Technical aspects and early clinical outcome. Journal of Endovascular Therapy. 2000;7(2):79-91

[11] Tagalakis V, Patenaude V, Kahn SR, Suissa S. Incidence of and mortality from venous thromboembolism in a real-world population: The Q-VTE study cohort. The American Journal of Medicine. 2013;**126**(9):832-e13

[12] Konstantinides SV, Barco S, Lankeit M, Meyer G. Management of pulmonary embolism: An update. Journal of the American College of Cardiology. 2016;**67**(8):976-990

[13] Konstantinides SV, Torbicki A, Agnelli G, et al. 2014 ESC guidelines on the diagnosis and management of acute pulmonary embolism. European Heart Journal. 2014;**35**(3033-69):3069a-3069k

[14] Engelberger RP, Kucher N. Ultrasound-assisted thrombolysis for acute pulmonary embolism: A systematic review. European Heart Journal. 2014;**35**:758-764

[15] Streiff MB. Vena caval filters: A comprehensive review. Blood, The

Journal of the American Society of Hematology. 2000;**95**(12):3669-3677

[16] Bauersachs RM. Clinical presentation of deep vein thrombosis and pulmonary embolism. Best Practice & Research Clinical Haematology. 2012;**25**(3):243-251

[17] Tapson VF. Acute pulmonary embolism. Cardiology Clinics. 2004;**22**(3):353-365

[18] Stein PD, Woodard PK, Weg JG, Wakefield TW, Tapson VF, Sostman HD, et al. Diagnostic pathways in acute pulmonary embolism: Recommendations of the PIOPED II investigators. The American Journal of Medicine. 2006;**119**(12):1048-1055

[19] Kline JA, Miller DW. Risk stratification for acute pulmonary embolism. Journal of the National Comprehensive Cancer Network. 2011;**9**(7):800-810

[20] Goldhaber SZ. Echocardiography in the management of pulmonary embolism. Annals of Internal Medicine. 2002;**136**(9):691-700

[21] Moumneh T, Wells PS, Miranda S. Risk stratification of pulmonary embolism. Critical Care Clinics. 2020;**36**(3):437-448

[22] Baram M, Awsare B, Merli G. Pulmonary embolism in intensive care units. Critical Care Clinics. 2020;**36**(3):427-435

[23] Kearon C, Kahn SR, Agnelli G, Goldhaber S, Raskob GE, Comerota AJ. Antithrombotic therapy for venous thromboembolic disease: American College of Chest Physicians evidence-based clinical practice guidelines. Chest. 2008;**133**(6):454S-545S

[24] Stein PD, Fowler SE, Goodman LR, Gottschalk A, Hales CA, Hull RD, et al. Multidetector computed tomography for acute pulmonary embolism. New England Journal of Medicine. 2006;**354**(22):2317-2327

[25] Tapson VF, Davidson CJ, Kisslo KB, Stack RS. Rapid visualization of massive pulmonary emboli utilizing intravascular ultrasound. Chest. 1994;**105**(3):888-890

[26] Frémont B, Pacouret G, Jacobi D, Puglisi R, Charbonnier B, de Labriolle A. Prognostic value of echocardiographic right/left ventricular end-diastolic diameter ratio in patients with acute pulmonary embolism: Results from a monocenter registry of 1,416 patients. Chest. 2008;**133**(2):358-362

[27] Piazza G, Goldhaber SZ. Management of sub-massive pulmonary embolism. Circulation. 2010;**122**:1124-1129

[28] Mookadam F, Jiamsripong P, Goel R, Warsame TA, Emani UR, Khandheria BK. Critical appraisal on the utility of echocardiography in the management of acute pulmonary embolism. Cardiology in Review. 2010;**18**:29-37. DOI: 10.1097/CRD.0b013e3181c09443

[29] Serafini O, Greco F, Misuraca G, Chiatto M, Buffon A. Echocardiography in the diagnostic and prognostic evaluation of thromboembolic pulmonary hypertension. Archives for Chest Disease. 2005;**64**:116-123

[30] Ruohoniemi DM, Sista AK. Interventional radiology therapy: Inferior vena cava filter and catheter-based therapies. Critical Care Clinics. 2020;**36**(3):481-495

[31] Pulido T, Aranda A, Zevallos MA, Bautista E, Martínez-Guerra ML,

Santos LE, et al. Pulmonary embolism as a cause of death in patients with heart disease: An autopsy study. Chest. 2006;**129**(5):1282-1287

[32] Kuo WT. Endovascular therapy for acute pulmonary embolism. Journal of Vascular and Interventional Radiology. 2012;**23**(2):167-179

[33] Kuo WT, Gould MK, Louie JD, Rosenberg JK, Sze DY, Hofmann LV. Catheter-directed therapy for the treatment of massive pulmonary embolism: Systematic review and meta-analysis of modern techniques. Journal of Vascular and Interventional Radiology. 2009;**20**(11):1431-1440

[34] Uflacker R, Strange C, Vujic I. Massive pulmonary embolism: Preliminary results of treatment with the Amplatz thrombectomy device. Journal of Vascular and Interventional Radiology. 1996;**7**(4):519-528

[35] Schmitz-Rode T, Kilbinger M, Günther RW. Simulated flow pattern in massive pulmonary embolism: Significance for selective intrapulmonary thrombolysis. Cardiovascular and Interventional Radiology. 1998;**21**:199-204

[36] Heit JA, Spencer FA, White RH. The epidemiology of venous thromboembolism. Journal of Thrombosis and Thrombolysis. 2016;**41**:3-14

[37] Bernardi E, Camporese G, Büller HR, Siragusa S, Imberti D, Berchio A, et al. Serial 2-point ultrasonography plus D-dimer vs whole-leg color-coded Doppler ultrasonography for diagnosing suspected symptomatic deep vein thrombosis: A randomized controlled trial. JAMA. 2008;**300**(14):1653-1659

[38] Kocakoc E. Detection of deep vein thrombosis with Doppler sonography. Journal of Thrombosis and Thrombolysis. 2008;**26**:159-160

[39] Sumner DS, Lambeth A. Reliability of Doppler ultrasound in the diagnosis of acute venous thrombosis both above and below the knee. The American Journal of Surgery. 1979;**138**(2):205-210

[40] Fortes VB, Rollo HA, Fortes AT Jr, Sobreira MDL, Santos FC, Giannini M, et al. et al. Clinical prediction model in the diagnosis of deep vein thrombosis of the thrombosis of the lower limbs. Brazilian Vascular Journal. 2007;**6**:7-16

[41] Onuoha CU. Phlegmasia cerulea dolens: A rare clinical presentation. The American Journal of Medicine. 2015;**128**(9):e27-e28

[42] Aydemir B, Hoyle C, Hakmeh W. Phlegmasia cerulea dolens causing compartment syndrome. The American Journal of Emergency Medicine. 2022;**61**:234-2e1

[43] Chinsakchai K, Ten Duis K, Moll FL, De Borst GJ. Trends in management of phlegmasia cerulea dolens. Vascular and Endovascular Surgery. 2011;**45**(1):5-14

[44] Suciadi LP, Aristo AN. Phlegmasia Alba Dolens Complicating Rhabdomyolysis. Cureus. 24 Mar 2021;**13**(3):e14080. DOI: 10.7759/cureus.14080

[45] Raju S, Ward M Jr, Davis M. Relative importance of iliac vein obstruction in patients with post-thrombotic femoral vein occlusion. Journal of Vascular Surgery: Venous and Lymphatic Disorders. 2015;**3**(2):161-167

[46] Pouncey AL, Gwozdz AM, Johnson OW, Silickas J, Saha P, Thulasidasan N, et al. AngioJet pharmacomechanical thrombectomy and catheter directed thrombolysis vs.

catheter directed thrombolysis alone for the treatment of iliofemoral deep vein thrombosis: A single Centre retrospective cohort study. European Journal of Vascular and Endovascular Surgery. 2020;**60**(4):578-585

[47] Aburahma AF, Robinson PA, Boland JP. Clinical, hemodynamic, and anatomic predictors of long-term outcome of lower extremity venovenous bypasses. Journal of Vascular Surgery. 1991;**14**(5):635-644

[48] Delis KT, Bountouroglou D, Mansfield AO. Venous claudication in iliofemoral thrombosis: Long-term effects on venous hemodynamics, clinical status, and quality of life. Annals of Surgery. 2004;**239**(1):118-126

[49] Subbiah R, Aggarwal V, Zhao H, Kolluri R, Chatterjee S, Bashir R. Effect of compression stockings on post thrombotic syndrome in patients with deep vein thrombosis: A meta-analysis of randomised controlled trials. The Lancet Haematology. 2016;**3**(6):e293-e300

[50] Delis KT, Bjarnason H, Wennberg PW, Rooke TW, Gloviczki P. Successful iliac vein and inferior vena cava stenting ameliorates venous claudication and improves venous outflow, calf muscle pump function, and clinical status in post-thrombotic syndrome. Annals of Surgery. 2007;**245**(1):130-139

[51] Harris JP, Kidd J, Burnett A, Halliday P, May J. Patency of femorofemoral venous crossover grafts assessed by duplex scanning and phlebography. Journal of Vascular Surgery. 1988;**8**(6):679-682

[52] Bergan JJ, Yao JS. Venous reconstructive surgery. In: Vascular Surgical Techniques. Butterworth-Heinemann; 1984. pp. 275-283

[53] Sandri GDA. Endovascular treatment of chronic venous obstructions of the iliocaval segment. Brazilian Vascular Journal. 2011;**10**:137-144

[54] Dronkers CEA, Mol GC, Maraziti G, Van De Ree MA, Huisman MV, Becattini C, et al. Predicting post-thrombotic syndrome with ultrasonographic follow-up after deep vein thrombosis: A systematic review and meta-analysis. Thrombosis and Haemostasis. 2018;**118**(08):1428-1438

[55] Schleimer K, Barbati ME, Grommes J, Hoeft K, Toonder IM, Wittens CH, et al. Update on diagnosis and treatment strategies in patients with post-thrombotic syndrome due to chronic venous obstruction and role of endovenous recanalization. Journal of Vascular Surgery: Venous and Lymphatic Disorders. 2019;**7**(4):592-600

[56] Jayaraj A, Raju S. Three-dimensional computed tomography venogram enables accurate diagnosis and treatment of patients presenting with symptomatic chronic iliofemoral venous obstruction. Journal of Vascular Surgery: Venous and Lymphatic Disorders. 2021;**9**(1):73-80

[57] Gagne PJ, Tahara RW, Fastabend CP, Dzieciuchowicz L, Marston W, Vedantham S, et al. Venography versus intravascular ultrasound for diagnosing and treating iliofemoral vein obstruction. Journal of Vascular Surgery: Venous and Lymphatic Disorders. 2017;**5**(5):678-687

[58] Neglén P, Raju S. Intravascular ultrasound scan evaluation of the obstructed vein. Journal of Vascular Surgery. 2002;**35**(4):694-700

[59] Fonseca AG, Amado M. Thrombophilias: Importance of their study in thromboembolic pathology. Internal Medicine. 2008;**15**(4):284-290

[60] Razavi MK, Black S, Gagne P, Chiacchierini R, Nicolini P, Marston W, et al. Pivotal study of endovenous stent placement for symptomatic iliofemoral venous obstruction. Circulation: Cardiovascular Interventions. 2019;**12**(12):e008268

[61] Williams ZF, Dillavou ED. A systematic review of venous stents for iliac and venacaval occlusive disease. Journal of Vascular Surgery: Venous and Lymphatic Disorders. 2020;**8**(1):145-153

[62] Grøtta O, Enden T, Sandbæk G, Gjerdalen GF, Slagsvold CE, Bay D, et al. Infrainguinal inflow assessment and endovenous stent placement in iliofemoral post-thrombotic obstructions. CVIR Endovascular. 2018;**1**:1-9

[63] Rizvi SA, Ascher E, Hingorani A, Marks N. Stent patency in patients with advanced chronic venous disease and nonthrombotic iliac vein lesions. Journal of Vascular Surgery: Venous and Lymphatic Disorders. 2018;**6**(4): 457-463

[64] Decousus H, Leizorovicz A, Parent F, Page Y, Tardy B, Girard P, et al. A clinical trial of vena caval filters in the prevention of pulmonary embolism in patients with proximal deep-vein thrombosis. New England Journal of Medicine. 1998;**338**(7):409-416

[65] Athanasoulis CA, Kaufman JA, Halpern EF, Waltman AC, Geller SC, Fan CM. Inferior vena caval filters: Review of a 26-year single-center clinical experience. Radiology. 2000;**216**(1):54-66

[66] Trendelenburg F. On the operation of embolism of the pulmonary artery. DMW-Deutsche Medizinische Wochenschrift. 1908;**34**(27):1172-1174

[67] Goldhaber SZ, Buring JE, Lipnick RJ, Stubblefield F, Hennekens CH. Interruption of the inferior vena cava by clip or filter. The American Journal of Medicine. 1984;**76**(3):512-516

[68] Dodson MG, Mobin-Uddin K, O'Leary JA. Intracaval umbrella-filter for prevention of recurrent pulmonary embolism. Southern Medical Journal. 1971;**64**(8):1017-1018

[69] De Gregorio MA. Inferior vena cava filter update. Archivos de Bronconeumología (English Edition). 2004;**40**(5):193-195

[70] Greenfield LJ, McCurdy JR, Brown PP, Elkins RC. A new intracaval filter permitting continued flow and resolution of emboli. Surgery. 1973;**73**(4):599-606

[71] Goodman LR, Stein PD, Matta F, Sostman HD, Wakefield TW, Woodard PK, et al. CT venography and compression sonography are diagnostically equivalent: Data from PIOPED II. American Journal of Roentgenology. 2007;**189**(5):1071-1076

[72] Gottschalk A, Stein PD, Goodman LR, Sostman HD. Overview of prospective investigation of pulmonary embolism diagnosis II. In: Seminars in Nuclear Medicine. Vol. 32(3). WB Saunders; 2002. pp. 173-182